MASQUERADE SYNDROME IN OPHTHALMOLOGY

A Clinical Handbook of the Great Imitators of the Eye

When the eye lies, the clinician must listen harder.

SuVi Eye Hospital and Lasik Laser Centre, Kota

First Edition · 2026

FIRST EDITION · 2026

MASQUERADE SYNDROME IN OPHTHALMOLOGY

A Clinical Handbook of the Great Imitators of the Eye

Edited by the Clinical Editorial Board

SuVi Eye Hospital and Lasik Laser Centre, Kota

Kota, Rajasthan, India

This handbook is intended as an educational reference for qualified ophthalmologists and ophthalmic trainees. It is not a substitute for clinical judgement or specialist consultation.

DEDICATION

For the Clinicians Who Look Twice

To every ophthalmologist who has ever stared at a slit lamp at midnight, wondering whether what looks like inflammation is something else entirely- this book is for you, and for the patients whose eyes we promise to look at twice.

FOREWORD

On Disguise and Vigilance

In thirty years of practice, I have learned one humbling lesson: the eye is honest, but it is not always plain-spoken. It rarely tells us, on the first visit, what it is suffering from. The disciplines of uveitis and ocular oncology meet, again and again, in a clinical clearing called the masquerade the place where what we see is not what we are treating. Masquerades are the great teachers of ophthalmology. They demand humility from the confident clinician and confidence from the humble one. They reward those who listen, look, and look again.

This handbook is for the ophthalmologist working anywhere in the academic centre, in the busy district hospital, and in the rural eye-care camp. It is meant to live on the desk between the slit lamp and the consulting chair, opened when something does not quite fit the textbook. It is meant to be reread, annotated, and argued with. Each chapter is short enough to read between two appointments and detailed enough to inform a complex decision.

The world has moved on from Theodore's 1967 description of the masquerade syndrome in a single clinical scenario. Today we know that the term covers a constellation of neoplastic, infectious, autoimmune, drug-induced and developmental conditions, each able to imitate intraocular inflammation. The diagnostic toolbox has grown — molecular cytology, high-resolution imaging, immunophenotyping — but the most powerful instrument remains the clinician's mind, asking the same disciplined question: what else could this be?

We hope this handbook helps you ask that question, and answer it, with greater confidence.

— SuVi Eye Hospital and Lasik Laser Centre, Kota

CONTENTS

Table of Contents

Foreword · Prologue · Three Sections · Twelve Chapters · Epilogue · References

SECTION I

Foundations of Masquerade Syndrome

SECTION II

Neoplastic Masquerades

SECTION III

Non-Neoplastic Masquerades

PROLOGUE

The Great Imitator

Every ophthalmologist remembers a case. Mine was a 72-year-old retired schoolteacher, referred for 'bilateral chronic intermediate uveitis, steroid-resistant'. She had been on topical, periocular and systemic corticosteroids for fourteen months. Her vitreous remained filled with cells; her vision continued to drift. On the third clinic visit, I noticed something subtle on her OCT — small hyper-reflective deposits at the level of the retinal pigment epithelium, the architecture of the outer retina disturbed in a way that did not obey the geometry of uveitis. A week later, the diagnostic vitrectomy returned with the answer no clinician wishes to read on a Friday afternoon: primary vitreoretinal lymphoma. The MRI showed cerebral involvement. Treatment changed entirely. The story did not end the way we wanted, but the diagnosis though late, gave her family the dignity of knowing.

I tell this story because it is not unusual. The literature suggests that between 5% and 20% of patients referred to tertiary uveitis services are eventually diagnosed with a masquerade syndrome. Among the elderly, the figure climbs higher. The reasons are familiar to every ophthalmologist: the eye is a small space; inflammation is a final common pathway; the temptation to escalate steroids is enormous; and the symptoms of malignancy or chronic infection often whisper before they shout.

The word 'masquerade' was chosen carefully when Theodore first used it in 1967. A masquerade is more than a disguise: it is a costume worn at a gathering, where the audience is expected to play along. The disease 'plays along' with our diagnostic categories until we look closely enough to lift the mask. Some masquerades — ocular syphilis, ocular tuberculosis, drug-induced uveitis can be unmasked by serology, history, or after a careful review of medications. Others primary vitreoretinal lymphoma, diffuse iris melanoma, retinoblastoma in the older child demand procedures that we must be willing to plan .

This book is a tour of the masquerade ball. It is divided into three sections — Foundations, Neoplastic Masquerades, and Non-Neoplastic Masquerades — twelve chapters in all. We start with the conceptual ground: what masquerade syndrome is, how it has evolved, and how to think systematically about a case that does not fit the script. We then walk into the world of neoplastic masquerades, where the costume is most often deadly and the stakes highest. We close with the rich landscape of non-neoplastic mimics — infectious, autoimmune, iatrogenic, developmental — each a reminder that the eye lives in conversation with the body and the medicine cabinet.

Throughout, we have tried to keep the writing close to the clinic. Figures are real eyes. Tables collect the kinds of facts you want at hand. Flowcharts capture the workflow you wish you had on the wall above your slit lamp. References, in Vancouver style, point to the literature you can consult after the patient leaves. Above all, we have tried to write a book that an ophthalmologist anywhere in the world — Kota or Cairo, São Paulo or Sydney — can read and recognise as a companion in the work we share.

If a single sentence summarises the spirit of this handbook, let it be this: when the eye stops responding to inflammation that was never inflammation in the first place, do not raise the dose. Raise the question.

SECTION I

Foundations of Masquerade Syndrome

The conceptual ground beneath the diagnostic art. This section establishes how the masquerade was named, why it matters, and the disciplined clinical thinking every ophthalmologist must rehearse before declaring a case 'uveitis'.

SECTION I · CHAPTER 01

Introduction and Historical Perspective

The Birth of a Diagnostic Idea

The word 'masquerade' arrived in the ophthalmic vocabulary almost as a metaphor. In 1967, Frederick Theodore described a conjunctival carcinoma that had been treated for years as chronic conjunctivitis. He called it a masquerade — a disease pretending to be something more familiar — and the word stayed. Over the next half century the term has expanded well beyond its original origin

CHAPTER 01

Introduction and Historical Perspective

The Birth of a Diagnostic Idea

The word 'masquerade' arrived in the ophthalmic vocabulary almost as a metaphor. In 1967, Frederick Theodore described a conjunctival carcinoma that had been treated for years as chronic conjunctivitis. He called it a masquerade — a disease pretending to be something more familiar — and the word stayed. Over the next half century the term has expanded well beyond its original ocular surface description to encompass any condition that imitates intraocular inflammation. It now covers entities as different as primary vitreoretinal lymphoma and rifabutin-induced uveitis, with the only common thread being the disguise itself.[1,2]

1.1 Theodore's original description

Theodore's 1967 paper described an elderly woman with a chronic, unilateral, follicular conjunctivitis that had been treated with topical antibiotics and corticosteroids for almost two years before a biopsy revealed an invasive squamous cell carcinoma of the conjunctiva.[1] The case was, at the time, a warning more than a category. Theodore proposed that 'unusual conjunctival lesions that mimic chronic inflammation' deserved a dedicated name. He chose the word 'masquerade' because the disease was a costume worn at a clinical ball — and because, like every good costume, it was both convincing and removable.

Within a decade, the concept had migrated inward. Ophthalmologists began to describe intraocular conditions — primarily lymphomas and metastatic carcinomas that presented as 'chronic refractory uveitis'. By 1989, Rothova and colleagues were able to publish a case series of 56 patients with intraocular masquerade syndromes, classifying them broadly into neoplastic and non-neoplastic groups.[3] The category has grown ever since, but the fundamental clinical lesson has not changed.

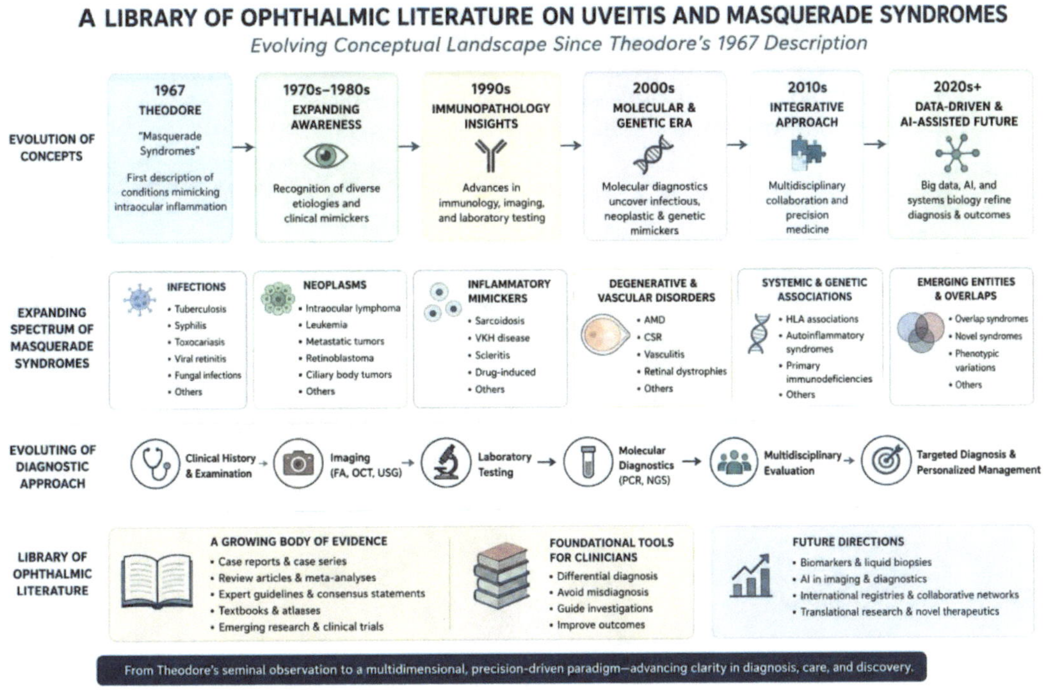

Figure 1.1 — A library of ophthalmic literature on uveitis and masquerade syndromes, illustrating the evolving conceptual landscape since Theodore's 1967 description.

1.2 Why the word still matters

Words shape practice. By calling a class of diseases 'masquerade syndromes', ophthalmologists give themselves permission to suspect them. The word warns the trainee that some patients with apparent uveitis do not, in fact, have uveitis. It encourages the senior clinician to revisit a diagnosis when the treatment is not working. It justifies to the patient, the family and the insurance system — the cost of a diagnostic vitrectomy, the MRI, the interdisciplinary consultation.

It also names a humility. Few diagnostic categories in ophthalmology are so openly an admission that we will, sometimes, be wrong. The masquerade reminds us that pattern recognition is not the same as truth, and that the costume of inflammation is one that many diseases can wear.

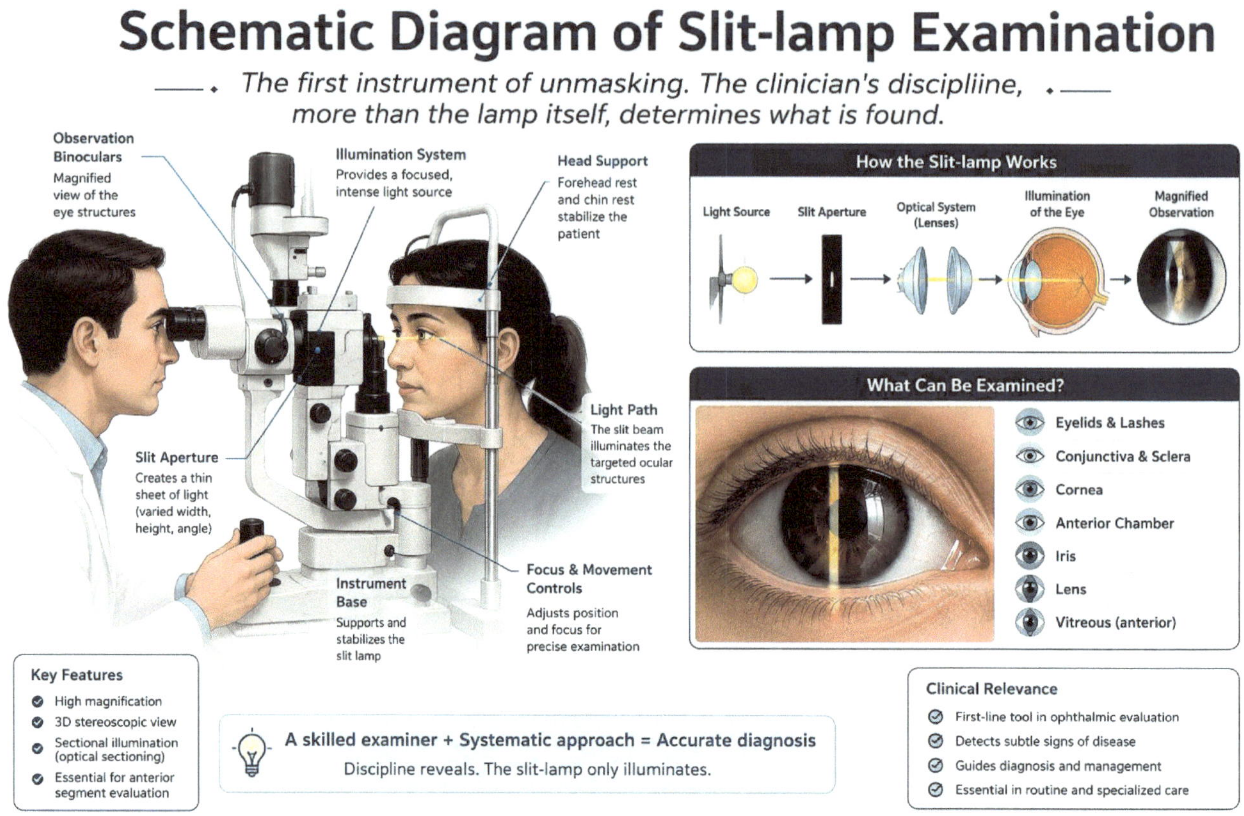

Figure 1.1 — Slit-lamp examination is the first instrument of unmasking. The clinician's discipline, more than the lamp itself, determines what is found.

1.3 Magnitude of the problem

Quantifying masquerade syndromes is difficult precisely because, by definition, they are initially misdiagnosed. The most cited series is that of Rothova et al., who found that 5% of patients referred to a tertiary uveitis service had a masquerade syndrome.[3] Among patients over 60 years of age, the figure rises to between 10% and 20% in some series. Primary vitreoretinal lymphoma alone has an estimated incidence of 0.046 per 100,000 person-years but represents a disproportionate share of the missed diagnoses in older adults with steroid-resistant vitritis.[5]

Beyond raw numbers, the consequences of missed masquerades are large. A late diagnosis of intraocular lymphoma is associated with worse visual outcomes and a higher risk of CNS spread. A late diagnosis of ocular syphilis can permit irreversible optic atrophy. A retained intraocular foreign body misread as anterior uveitis can incite siderosis. The cost — visual and human — is the reason the category exists at all.

TABLE 1.1

Landmark publications in masquerade syndrome

Year	Author / Reference	Contribution
1967	Theodore	Coined the term 'masquerade syndrome' for conjunctival lesions mimicking chronic inflammation.
1989	Read et al.	Classification of intraocular masquerades into neoplastic and non-neoplastic groups.
1995	Chan et al., NEI	IL-10/IL-6 cytokine ratio in vitreous as a biomarker for PVRL.
2014	Chan et al.	International Primary CNS Lymphoma Collaborative Group consensus on diagnosis.
2015	Bonzheim et al.	MYD88 L265P mutation as a molecular diagnostic for vitreoretinal lymphoma.
2019	Touhami et al.	Updated diagnostic algorithm integrating clinical, imaging and molecular criteria.

1.4 How this handbook is organised

We have divided the handbook into three sections. Section I (the present section) covers Foundations: the conceptual ground, the working classification, the clinical approach, and the diagnostic toolbox. Section II is devoted to Neoplastic Masquerades, beginning with primary vitreoretinal lymphoma — the archetype — and continuing through metastatic disease, uveal and iris tumours, and ocular surface and paediatric tumours. Section III covers Non-Neoplastic Masquerades, including infectious mimics (with particular attention to ocular syphilis and tuberculosis), autoimmune and granulomatous disease, drug-induced and iatrogenic masquerades, and the rare or paediatric entities every clinician will encounter.

Each chapter is short by design. The aim is not encyclopaedic completeness but clinical utility — a book that fits beside the slit lamp.

CLINICAL PEARLS

- The word 'masquerade' was coined by Theodore in 1967 to describe a conjunctival carcinoma misdiagnosed as conjunctivitis. It has since expanded to all conditions that mimic intraocular inflammation.
- Between 5% and 20% of patients in tertiary uveitis services have a masquerade syndrome; the figure rises with age.
- The category exists to give clinicians permission to suspect, not just to recognise, atypical disease.
- Late diagnosis of a masquerade can be lethal in neoplastic disease and blinding in infectious disease.

KEY POINTS

1. Theodore (1967) introduced the term in the context of a conjunctival carcinoma.
2. The term now encompasses neoplastic, infectious, autoimmune, drug-induced and developmental disease that mimics uveitis.
3. Masquerade syndromes are an act of clinical humility as much as a diagnostic category.
4. Pattern recognition is necessary but not sufficient; vigilance for atypical features is the daily practice.

SECTION I · CHAPTER 02

Classification, Epidemiology, and Pathophysiology

Anatomy of a Disguise

If Chapter 1 named the masquerade, Chapter 2 maps its territory. Any clinician who has worked through a tertiary uvea clinic will recognise the variety: a 72-year-old with vitritis that turns out to be lymphoma; a 28-year-old with iritis whose serum reveals syphilis; a 6-year-old with leukocoria whose 'uveitis' is in fact retinoblastoma. To navigate that variety, we need a w…

Figure 2.2 — Diagnostic workflow visualised in a clinical setting. Pattern recognition across age, laterality, and treatment response forms the backbone of suspicion.

CHAPTER 02

Classification, Epidemiology, and Pathophysiology

Anatomy of a Disguise

If Chapter 1 named the masquerade, Chapter 2 maps its territory. Any clinician who has worked through a tertiary uveitis clinic will recognise the variety: a 72-year-old with vitritis that turns out to be lymphoma; a 28-year-old with iritis whose serum reveals syphilis; a 6-year-old with leukocoria whose 'uveitis' is in fact retinoblastoma. To navigate that variety, we need a working classification, an honest sense of epidemiology, and a mechanistic understanding of how disguise becomes possible.[3,11]

2.1 A working classification

Masquerade syndromes are most usefully classified by aetiology. Neoplastic masquerades subdivide into primary intraocular (PVRL, uveal melanoma, iris melanoma, retinoblastoma) and metastatic or systemic (choroidal metastasis, leukaemia, paraneoplastic retinopathies).[2,17] Non-neoplastic masquerades subdivide into infectious, autoimmune/granulomatous, drug-induced/iatrogenic and developmental/structural categories. Each subcategory has its own epidemiology, its own diagnostic signature, and its own preferred therapy.

Some conditions span categories: a lymphoma may be both primary (PVRL) and systemic; an immune-checkpoint inhibitor may induce VKH-like disease that behaves like an autoimmune masquerade although the mechanism is iatrogenic. The clinician's task is to place each patient on this map and use the geography to guide the workup.

TABLE 2.1

Working classification of intraocular masquerade syndromes

Category	Representative Entities
Neoplastic — primary intraocular	Primary vitreoretinal lymphoma, uveal melanoma, diffuse iris melanoma, retinoblastoma
Neoplastic — metastatic / systemic	Choroidal metastasis (breast, lung), leukaemia, systemic lymphoma, paraneoplastic retinopathies
Infectious	Ocular syphilis, ocular tuberculosis, viral retinitis, endogenous endophthalmitis, Whipple disease
Autoimmune / granulomatous	Sarcoidosis, IgG4-related disease, granulomatosis with polyangiitis, Behçet's, VKH
Drug-induced / iatrogenic	Rifabutin, cidofovir, MEK/BRAF inhibitors, checkpoint inhibitors, retained IOFB, silicone oil
Developmental / structural	Persistent fetal vasculature, Coats disease, juvenile retinoschisis, FEVR

2.2 Global epidemiology

The epidemiology of masquerade syndromes mirrors the epidemiology of the underlying disease. In high-income settings, neoplastic masquerades — particularly PVRL — dominate referral statistics from tertiary uveitis services. In low- and middle-income countries, infectious masquerades — tuberculosis, syphilis, endemic viral retinitides — feature more prominently.[31,34] Both pictures are changing. The global resurgence of syphilis since 2010, the rapid expansion of immune-checkpoint inhibitor use in oncology, and the ageing of the population in most regions all reshape the differential each year.

PVRL has an estimated annual incidence of 30 to 50 cases per 10 million people in Western series.[26] Choroidal metastasis is the most common intraocular malignancy in adults overall, with breast and lung primaries predominating.[17] Among children under three years old presenting with uveitis-like signs,

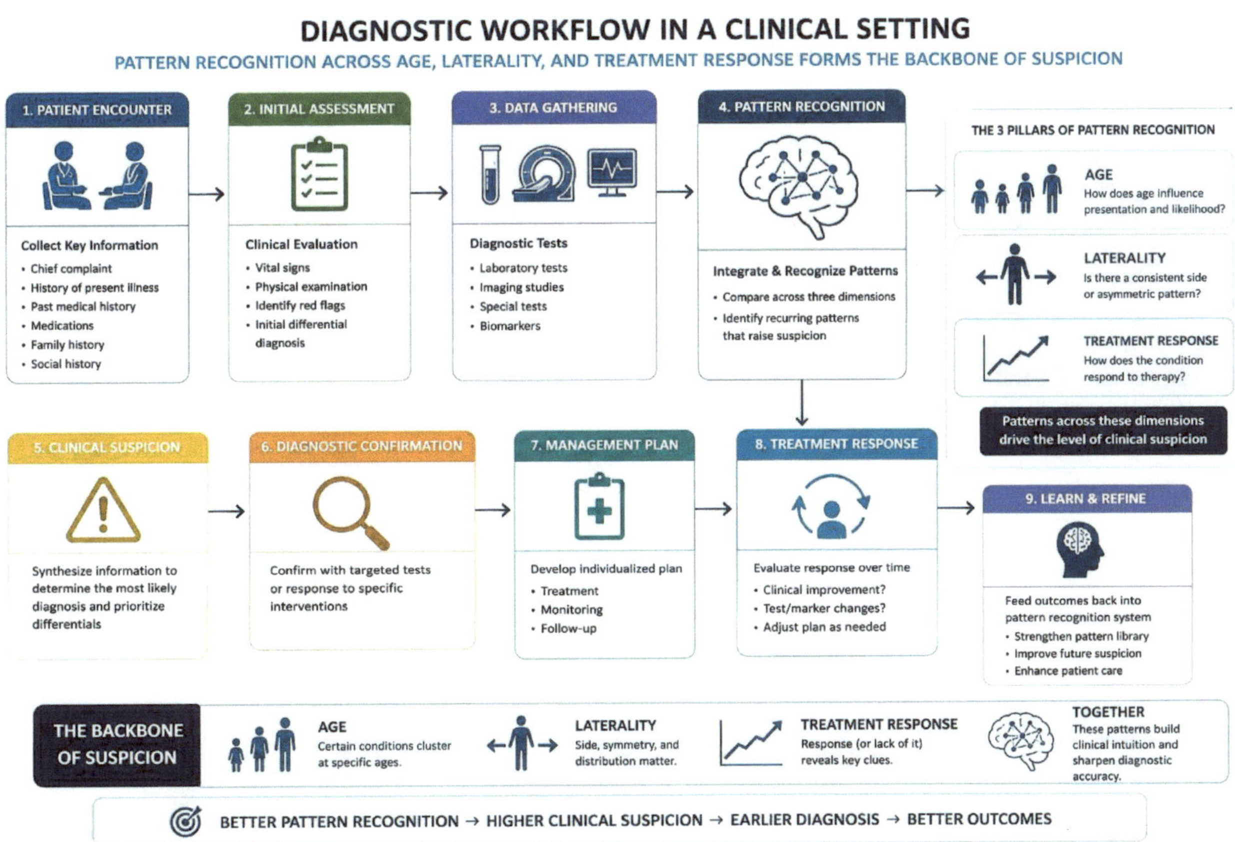

retinoblastoma must be excluded before any escalation of anti-inflammatory therapy.

Figure 2.2 — Diagnostic workflow visualised in a clinical setting. Pattern recognition across age, laterality, and treatment response forms the backbone of suspicion.

2.3 Pathophysiology of the disguise

Three broad mechanisms allow a non-uveitic disease to imitate uveitis. The first is direct cellular infiltration of intraocular tissues: lymphoma cells in the vitreous, metastatic carcinoma cells in the choroid, leukaemic cells in the retina or optic nerve. The cells produce a cellular reaction that, on slit-lamp examination, looks indistinguishable from inflammatory cells. The second mechanism is secondary inflammation: a tumour, foreign body or infection sets up an immune response that is genuine inflammation but is not the primary problem. Treating the inflammation without addressing the cause is therefore futile. The third mechanism is structural: a developmental or degenerative process (persistent fetal vasculature, retained intraocular foreign body, retinoschisis) produces a clinical picture that masquerades as uveitis despite having no primary inflammatory component.[71]

Understanding which mechanism is at work in a given case influences both the diagnostic approach (cytology for infiltration; serology for infection; imaging for structure) and the therapy. Mechanism-based reasoning, not appearance-based reasoning, is the heart of unmasking the masquerade.

2.4 Risk profiles to remember

Several patient phenotypes carry an elevated baseline risk of harbouring a masquerade. Adults over the age of 60 presenting with new vitritis are at particular risk of PVRL and must be investigated accordingly.[5,8] Patients with a personal history of any malignancy particularly breast, lung, gastrointestinal or haematological should be screened for choroidal metastasis at any new visual symptom.[17] Immunocompromised patients are at elevated risk of opportunistic viral retinitides, ocular syphilis, ocular tuberculosis and CMV retinitis presenting as panuveitis.[44,67] Children under three years old with persistent unilateral 'uveitis' must have retinoblastoma actively excluded.[47]

CLINICAL PEARLS

- Classify masquerades by aetiology: neoplastic vs non-neoplastic, and then by mechanism (infiltration, secondary inflammation, structural).
- Epidemiology shifts with geography and decade — track local infection prevalence and population age.
- Three patient profiles raise immediate suspicion: age >60 with vitritis, personal cancer history, immunocompromised.
- Children under 3 years with apparent uveitis require retinoblastoma exclusion before steroid escalation.

KEY POINTS

- Neoplastic and non-neoplastic categories each subdivide into clinically useful groups.
- Mechanism-based reasoning (infiltration, secondary inflammation, structural) drives diagnosis.
- Global epidemiology is changing — syphilis is rising, immune-checkpoint uveitis is new.
- Demographic phenotypes (age, comorbidity, immunity) are the strongest single risk modifiers.

SECTION I · CHAPTER 03

The Clinical Approach to a Suspected Masquerade

Listening to What the Eye Does Not Say

Most masquerades are diagnosed not at the microscope but at the slit lamp — by the clinician who took an unhurried history, examined the eye twice, and refused to settle for the easy label. This chapter is a practical guide to the moments where a masquerade should rise into the differential. It collects the red flags, the rhythm of follow-up, and the small habits of inspection ...

CHAPTER 03

The Clinical Approach to a Suspected Masquerade

Listening to What the Eye Does Not Say

Most masquerades are diagnosed not at the microscope but at the slit lamp — by the clinician who took an unhurried history, examined the eye twice, and refused to settle for the easy label. This chapter is a practical guide to the moments where a masquerade should rise into the differential. It collects the red flags, the rhythm of follow-up, and the small habits of inspection and listening that distinguish the clinician who finds a masquerade from the one who treats it for two years as refractory uveitis.[3,11]

3.1 History: what the textbook does not write down

The history of a suspected masquerade should always begin with three deliberately open questions. First: when did this start, and what made you come in today? The patient's narrative; particularly the trajectory of symptoms often reveals subacute features that pure uveitis lacks. Second: what other doctors have you seen and what treatments have you had? A history of steroid escalation without improvement, of paradoxical worsening, of drug switches that never quite worked, is a red flag in itself. Third: are you well in yourself? Constitutional symptoms — weight loss, fever, night sweats, lymphadenopathy must always be sought because they may be the first hint of a systemic process.

A drug history is essential. Rifabutin, bisphosphonates, MEK and BRAF inhibitors, Aromatase inhibitors and the immune-checkpoint inhibitors are all potent causes of drug-induced uveitis; identifying them changes management overnight.[43] Travel history matters for endemic infections; sexual history matters for syphilis; needle-stick history matters for viral retinitis. The questions are uncomfortable, but they are also short.

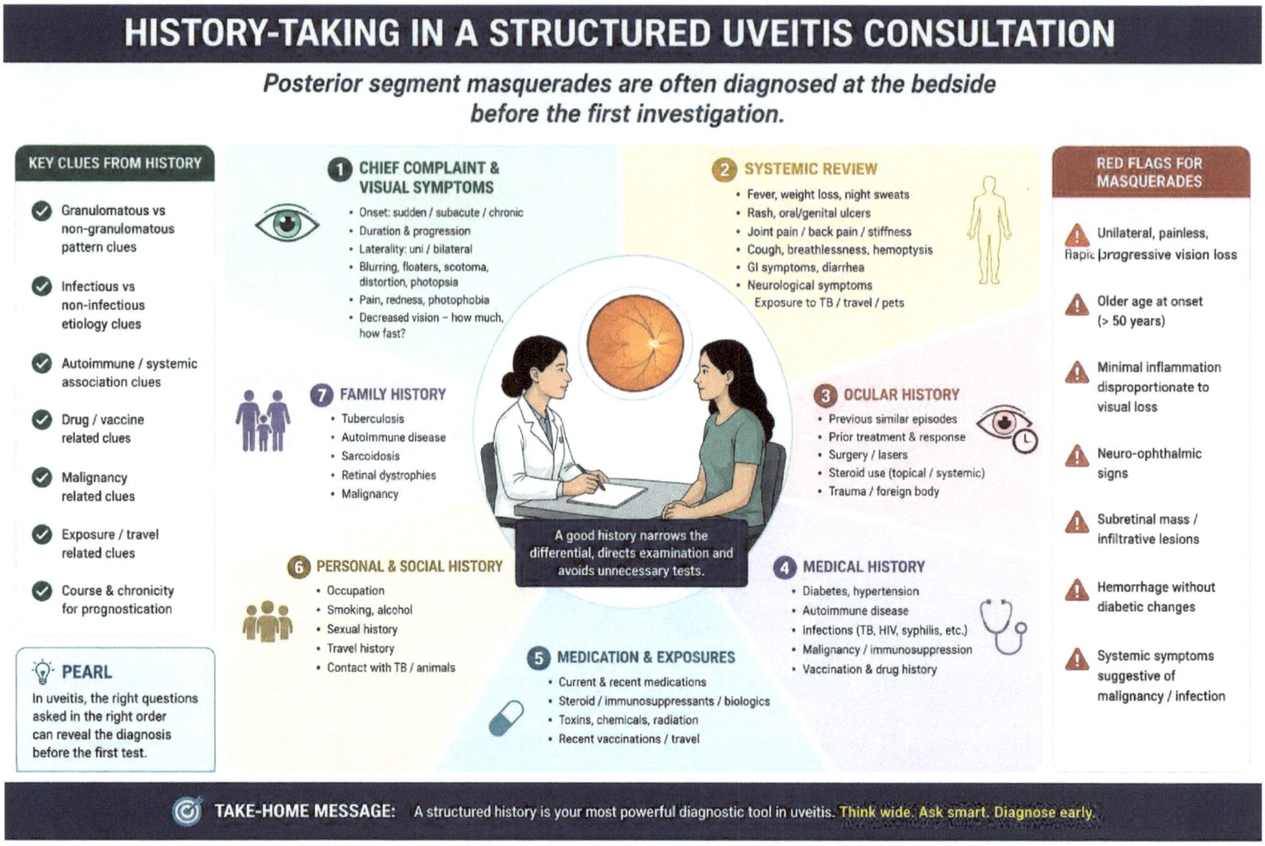
HISTORY-TAKING IN A STRUCTURED UVEITIS CONSULTATION
Posterior segment masquerades are often diagnosed at the bedside before the first investigation.
KEY CLUES FROM HISTORY
Granulomatous vs non-granulomatous pattern clues
Infectious vs non-infectious etiology clues
Autoimmune / systemic association clues
Drug / vaccine related clues
Malignancy related clues
Exposure / travel related clues
Course & chronicity for prognostication
PEARL
In uveitis, the right questions asked in the right order can reveal the diagnosis before the first test.
1 CHIEF COMPLAINT & VISUAL SYMPTOMS
Onset: sudden / subacute / chronic
Duration & progression
Laterality: uni / bilateral
Blurring, floaters, scotoma, distortion, photopsia
Pain, redness, photophobia
Decreased vision – how much, how fast?
2 SYSTEMIC REVIEW
Fever, weight loss, night sweats
Rash, oral/genital ulcers
Joint pain / back pain / stiffness
Cough, breathlessness, hemoptysis
GI symptoms, diarrhea
Neurological symptoms
Exposure to TB / travel / pets
3 OCULAR HISTORY
Previous similar episodes
Prior treatment & response
Surgery / lasers
Steroid use (topical / systemic)
Trauma / foreign body
4 MEDICAL HISTORY
Diabetes, hypertension
Autoimmune disease
Infections (TB, HIV, syphilis, etc.)
Malignancy / immunosuppression
Vaccination & drug history
5 MEDICATION & EXPOSURES
Current & recent medications
Steroid / immunosuppressants / biologics
Toxins, chemicals, radiation
Recent vaccinations / travel
6 PERSONAL & SOCIAL HISTORY
Occupation
Smoking, alcohol
Sexual history
Travel history
Contact with TB / animals
7 FAMILY HISTORY
Tuberculosis
Autoimmune disease
Sarcoidosis
Retinal dystrophies
Malignancy
A good history narrows the differential, directs examination and avoids unnecessary tests.
RED FLAGS FOR MASQUERADES
Unilateral, painless, rapid progressive vision loss
Older age at onset (> 50 years)
Minimal inflammation disproportionate to visual loss
Neuro-ophthalmic signs
Subretinal mass / infiltrative lesions
Hemorrhage without diabetic changes
Systemic symptoms suggestive of malignancy / infection
TAKE-HOME MESSAGE: A structured history is your most powerful diagnostic tool in uveitis. Think wide. Ask smart. Diagnose early.

Figure 3.1 — History-taking in a structured uveitis consultation: posterior segment masquerades are often diagnosed at the bedside before the first investigation.

3.2 Examination: looking twice

The slit-lamp examination of a possible masquerade should be slower than usual. Inspect the lid margin for sebaceous gland carcinoma masquerading as chronic blepharitis. Examine the conjunctiva in good light for the gelatinous vascular plaque of ocular surface squamous neoplasia or the salmon-pink infiltrate of conjunctival lymphoma.[21,22] Look at the iris under high magnification for heterochromia, sentinel vessels, or stromal nodules. Take the intraocular pressure carefully — diffuse iris melanoma, ghost cell glaucoma, and uveitic glaucoma each have characteristic pressure profiles. In the vitreous, watch for clumps and sheets of cells rather than the discrete individual cells of immune inflammation. In the fundus, search for subretinal yellow deposits, infiltrates with a 'leopard spotting' fluorescence pattern, and the geometric distortion of the outer retina that PVRL produces on OCT.[10,12]

When the examination is finished, document it. The single most useful habit of an uveitis clinician is to write what they saw in a way that another clinician — or the same clinician a year later — can compare to what they see now. Photographs and OCTs are essential. Drawings, oddly, are still underrated. The eye is the only organ we can see directly; the privilege deserves a record.

3.3 Red flags

Some clinical findings should make a masquerade suddenly probable rather than possible. We list them in Table 3.1 and apply them as a mental checklist at every uveitis follow-up. The most reliable red flag is treatment failure: an eye that does not behave as inflamed eyes are supposed to behave under appropriate therapy. The second most reliable is age — both the elderly patient and the very young child sit at the tails of the uveitis distribution. The third is the constellation of cell pattern, intraocular pressure, and posterior segment findings that, taken together, do not assemble into a recognisable uveitis pattern.

TABLE 3.1

Red flags suggesting a masquerade rather than primary uveitis

Domain	Red Flag
Demographic	Age >60 years (or <3 years), new-onset unilateral disease, history of malignancy
Clinical course	Steroid-resistant or steroid-dependent inflammation, paradoxical worsening on therapy
Examination	Out-of-proportion cells, vitreous clumps, subretinal yellow deposits, mass effect, sentinel vessels

Systemic	Constitutional symptoms, neurological signs, new lymphadenopathy, hepatosplenomegaly
Investigation	Serology negative, ACE/lysozyme negative, atypical OCT, MRI brain abnormalities
Response	Worsening on immunosuppression, relapse off therapy, atypical recurrence pattern

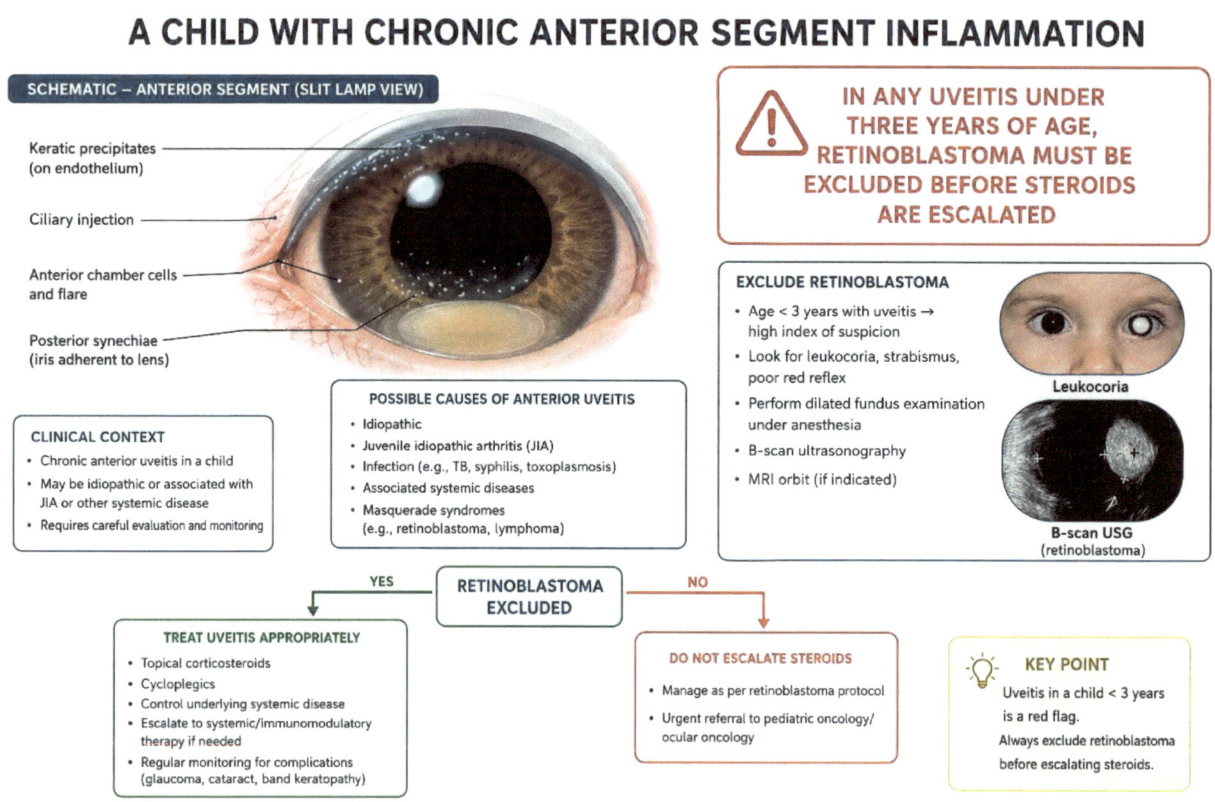

Figure 3.2 — A child with chronic anterior segment inflammation. In any uveitis under three years of age, retinoblastoma must be excluded before steroids are escalated.

3.4 A practical workflow

Flowchart 3.1 captures the workflow we use at SuVi Eye Hospital. It is deliberately modest in its first three steps: a careful history, a slow examination, and an honest list of red flags. Only after these have been completed do we order investigations. The discipline matters because investigation without a question is rarely useful in masquerade syndrome and the question is almost always best asked at the slit lamp.

FLOWCHART 3.1

Initial approach to suspected masquerade syndrome

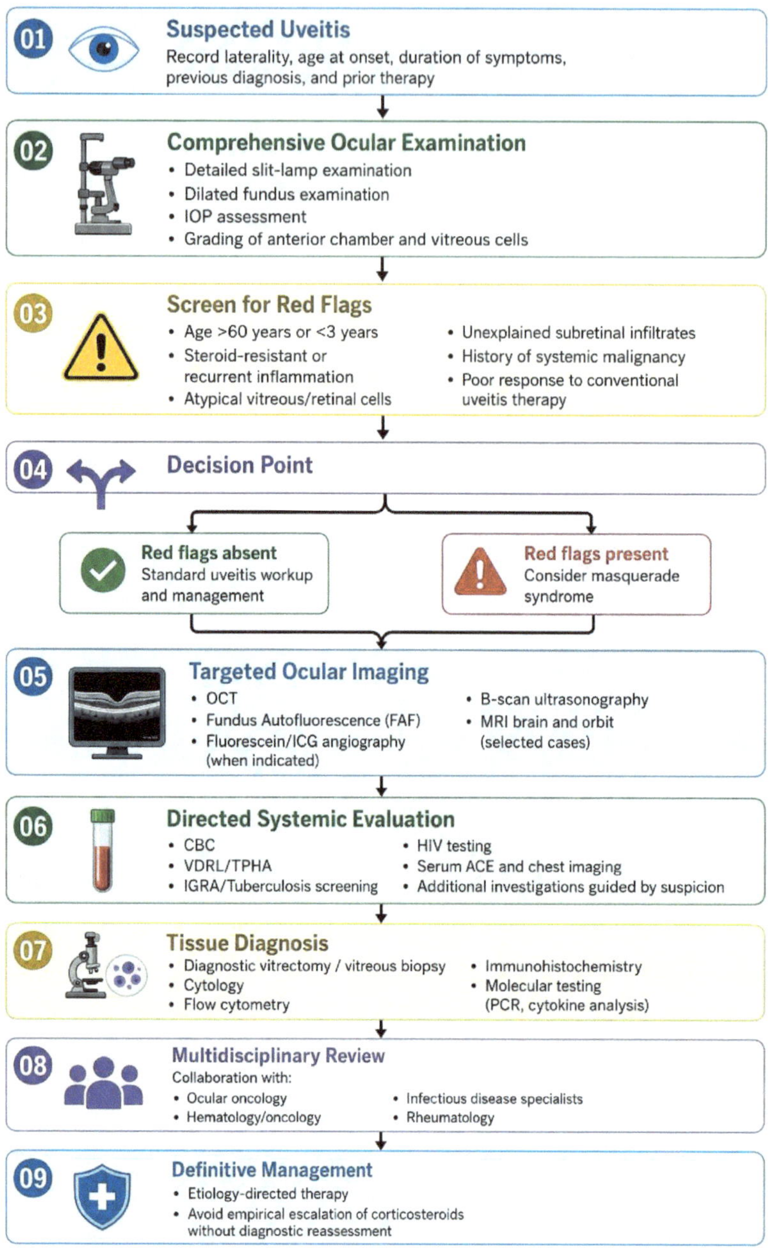

CLINICAL PEARLS

- Treatment failure is the most reliable red flag for masquerade syndrome.
- Document every uveitis examination with photographs and OCT; the next visit's diagnosis depends on it.
- Ask about systemic symptoms at every visit, not just the first.

- A drug review is part of the uveitis examination — not an afterthought.

KEY POINTS

- History, examination and red-flag recognition precede investigation.
- An eye that does not respond to appropriate therapy is, until proven otherwise, hiding a masquerade.
- Photographs, OCTs and structured notes are the diagnostic memory of the clinic.
- A standard workflow (history → examination → red flags → targeted investigation) reduces missed diagnoses.

SECTION I · CHAPTER 04

Diagnostic Modalities and Investigations

The Tools of Unmasking

Once the clinical suspicion is real, the diagnostic ecosystem decides the answer. This chapter is a brief tour of the tools — imaging, biopsy, molecular pathology, microbial PCR — that turn suspicion into diagnosis. None of them is independently sufficient. The diagnostic skill is in choosing, sequencing and interpreting them

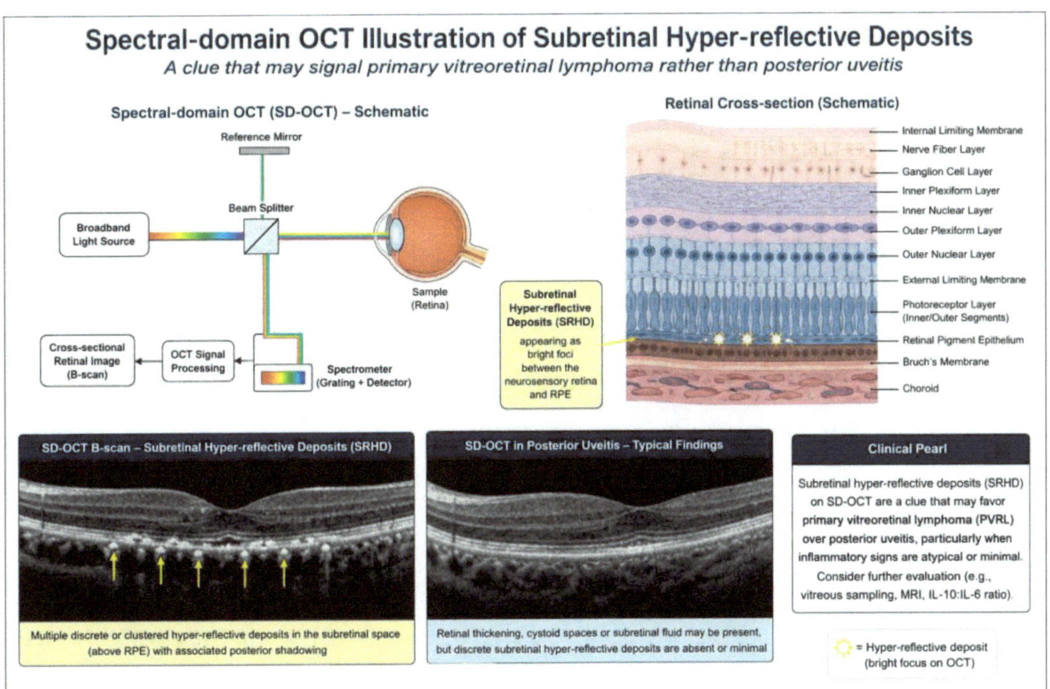

correctly, often in consultation with colleagues out…

Figure 4.1 — Spectral-domain OCT illustration of subretinal hyper-reflective deposits — a clue that may signal primary vitreoretinal lymphoma rather than posterior uveitis.

CHAPTER 04

Diagnostic Modalities and Investigations

The Tools of Unmasking

Once the clinical suspicion is real, the diagnostic ecosystem decides the answer. This chapter is a brief tour of the tools — imaging, biopsy, molecular pathology, microbial PCR — that turn suspicion into diagnosis. None of them is independently sufficient. The diagnostic skill is in choosing, sequencing and interpreting them correctly, often in consultation with colleagues outside ophthalmology.[12,13,55]

4.1 Imaging that talks back

Spectral-domain OCT is the workhorse of modern uveitis practice and the single most useful instrument for unmasking posterior segment masquerades. In PVRL, OCT typically shows hyper-reflective sub-RPE or subretinal deposits, with disturbance of the ellipsoid zone and undulations of the RPE. In choroidal metastasis, OCT shows characteristic dome elevation and overlying subretinal fluid. In paraneoplastic retinopathy, structural changes are often subtle, but the functional information from electroretinography seals the diagnosis.[10,12]

Fundus autofluorescence frequently reveals the 'leopard spotting' pattern of granular hyper- and hypo-autofluorescence in PVRL — a sign that is often more diagnostic than colour fundus photography itself. Fluorescein angiography demonstrates the staining patterns of choroidal infiltrates, and ICG angiography reveals the hypofluorescent dark spots characteristic of lymphomatous infiltration. B-scan ultrasound remains indispensable in eyes with media opacity and provides decisive measurements of choroidal masses, echo characteristics, and retained intraocular foreign bodies.[15,55]

TABLE 4.1

Diagnostic tools and their role in masquerade workup

Modality	Best for	Key finding
SD-OCT	Lymphoma, infiltrative lesions	Hyper-reflective sub-RPE / subretinal deposits, RPE undulations
Fundus autofluorescence	PVRL, paraneoplastic	Granular hyper- and hypo-autofluorescent areas ('leopard spotting')
FFA / ICG	Choroidal infiltration, vasculitis	Hypofluorescent dark spots on ICG; staining patterns on FFA
B-scan ultrasound	Posterior masses, IOFB	Vitreous opacities, mass dimensions, echo characteristics
MRI brain & orbit	PCNSL, optic nerve involvement	Periventricular enhancement, optic perineuritis
Vitreous biopsy + cytology	PVRL, leukaemia	Atypical lymphoid cells, IL-10:IL-6 > 1, MYD88 L265P
AC tap + PCR	Viral retinitis, toxoplasmosis	Detection of HSV/VZV/CMV DNA, T. gondii

4.2 Beyond the eye: MRI, CT and the systemic search

MRI of the brain and orbits is essential in any suspected primary vitreoretinal lymphoma, both for diagnosis and for staging. The characteristic finding is periventricular enhancement with subependymal spread, often bilateral and asymmetric.[14] A lumbar puncture with CSF cytology, flow cytometry and IL-10 measurement extends the staging beyond the eye. CT chest and abdomen is appropriate when systemic lymphoma is suspected and when the eye lesion may represent a metastatic deposit; HRCT chest is the screening imaging of choice for both sarcoidosis and tuberculosis when those diagnoses enter the differential.[29,30]

4.3 Diagnostic vitrectomy: when, why, how

Diagnostic vitrectomy is the procedure that most often turns suspicion of PVRL or other intravitreal masquerade into a diagnosis. Its yield depends on three principles, captured in Flowchart 4.1. First, the patient should be off systemic corticosteroids for at least two weeks where clinically safe, because lymphoid cells lyse rapidly under steroid pressure. Second, an undiluted vitreous sample should be collected at the start of the case before the infusion line is opened — this preserves cellular concentration. Third, the sample must reach the cytology laboratory within an hour, ideally in CytoLyt or equivalent fixative.[13,73]

Modern diagnostic vitrectomy delivers more than cytology. The sample can be sent for flow cytometry (clonality), IL-10/IL-6 ratio, MYD88 L265P mutation analysis (positive in ~70-90% of PVRL), and a broad microbial PCR panel covering HSV, VZV, CMV, EBV, T. gondii, and M. tuberculosis.[9,10,55,57] When the first sample is non-diagnostic but clinical suspicion remains, repeat biopsy is justified.

Figure 4.2 — Diagnostic vitrectomy in progress. Sample volume, handling, and rapid transit to the laboratory are the three commandments of cytological yield.

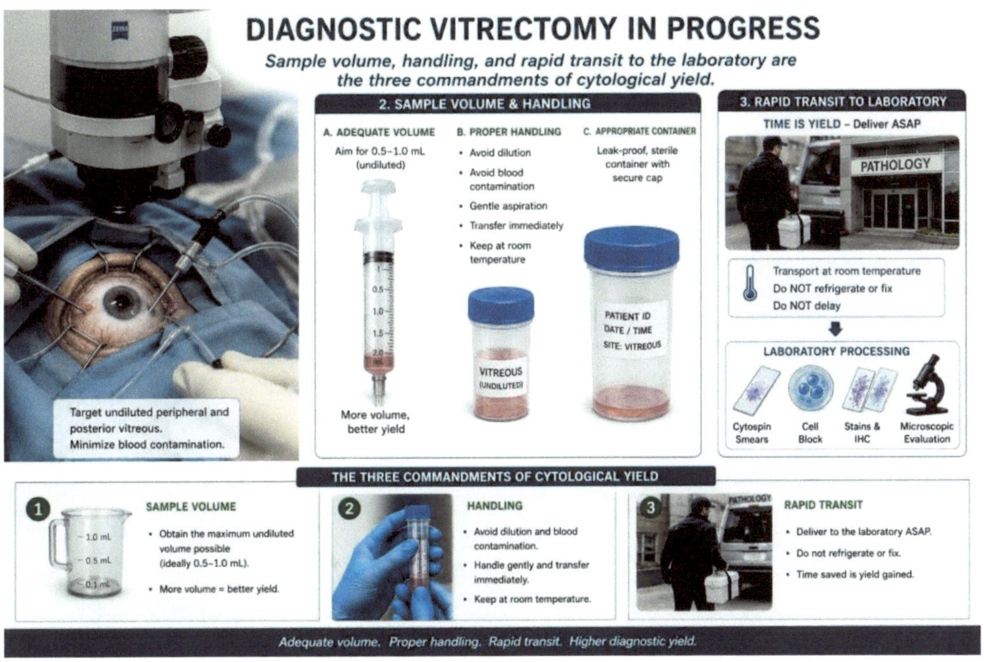

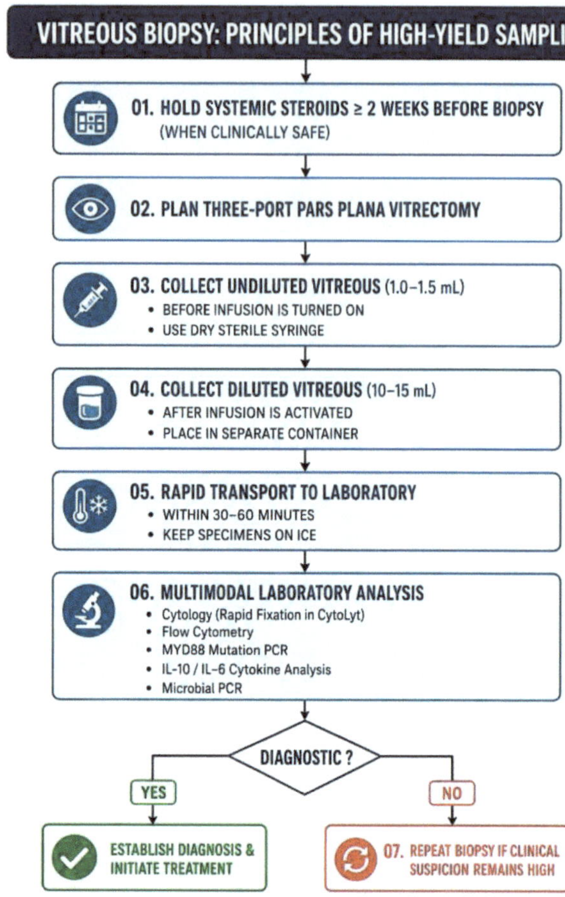

FLOWCHART 4.1

4.4 Molecular and microbial precision

Molecular tools have transformed masquerade diagnosis in the last decade. The MYD88 L265P mutation in PVRL is a near-pathognomonic marker present in the majority of cases.[10] Quantitative PCR for viral pathogens permits rapid identification of HSV, VZV, CMV and EBV from minimal aqueous samples, and 16S rRNA broad-range bacterial PCR can detect culture-negative bacterial endophthalmitis.[57,58,59] These tools are widely available in regional reference laboratories and should be used whenever the standard panel is non-diagnostic.

CLINICAL PEARLS

- Hold systemic steroids ≥2 weeks before diagnostic vitrectomy where safe — lymphoid cells lyse quickly.
- Collect undiluted vitreous (1.0–1.5 mL) at the start of vitrectomy, before opening the infusion.
- Send the sample for cytology, flow cytometry, IL-10:IL-6 ratio, MYD88 L265P and microbial PCR in parallel.
- Repeat biopsy when the first sample is non-diagnostic and suspicion persists.

KEY POINTS

- OCT, FAF, FFA, ICG and ultrasound each contribute a distinctive signature to the masquerade workup.
- MRI brain is essential in any suspected vitreoretinal lymphoma.
- Diagnostic vitrectomy is high-yield when its three procedural principles are respected.
- Molecular tools (MYD88, PCR panels) now seal diagnoses that cytology alone cannot.

SECTION II

Neoplastic Masquerades

Cancer wearing the costume of inflammation. From primary vitreoretinal lymphoma to choroidal metastasis and ocular surface neoplasia, this section maps the malignancies that the eye most often disguises and the windows through which we can see them clearly.

SECTION II · CHAPTER 05

Primary Vitreoretinal Lymphoma and CNS Lymphoma

The Lymphoma That Walks Behind the Iris

Primary vitreoretinal lymphoma (PVRL) is the masquerade by which all other intraocular masquerades are judged. It typically presents in adults over the age of 60 with bilateral but asymmetric vitritis, drifting vision, and a remarkable resistance to corticosteroid therapy. It is closely linked to primary central nervous system lymphoma (PCNSL): approximately 60-80% of patients ...

CHAPTER 05

Primary Vitreoretinal Lymphoma and CNS Lymphoma

The Lymphoma That Walks Behind the Iris

Primary vitreoretinal lymphoma (PVRL) is the masquerade by which all other intraocular masquerades are judged. It typically presents in adults over the age of 60 with bilateral but asymmetric vitritis, drifting vision, and a remarkable resistance to corticosteroid therapy. It is closely linked to primary central nervous system lymphoma (PCNSL): approximately 60-80% of patients with PVRL eventually develop CNS disease, and 15-25% of patients with PCNSL have ocular involvement at presentation.[5,8,11,14]

5.1 Clinical phenotype

The classic presentation is an older adult — most often in the seventh or eighth decade — with progressive painless visual loss, floaters, and a diffuse vitritis on examination. The vitreous cells of PVRL classically form clumps and sheets rather than the discrete cells of inflammatory uveitis. Posterior segment examination may show creamy yellow subretinal lesions, retinal pigment epithelium undulations, and on FAF a granular 'leopard spotting' pattern.[10,12] Vitreous cells may settle into characteristic 'aurora borealis' patterns when viewed on indirect ophthalmoscopy.

The clinical course is the most reliable diagnostic feature. PVRL typically improves transiently with corticosteroids and then relapses or worsens despite escalation. A waxing and waning course in an older adult with vitritis, particularly bilateral involvement, should prompt the workup described in this chapter.

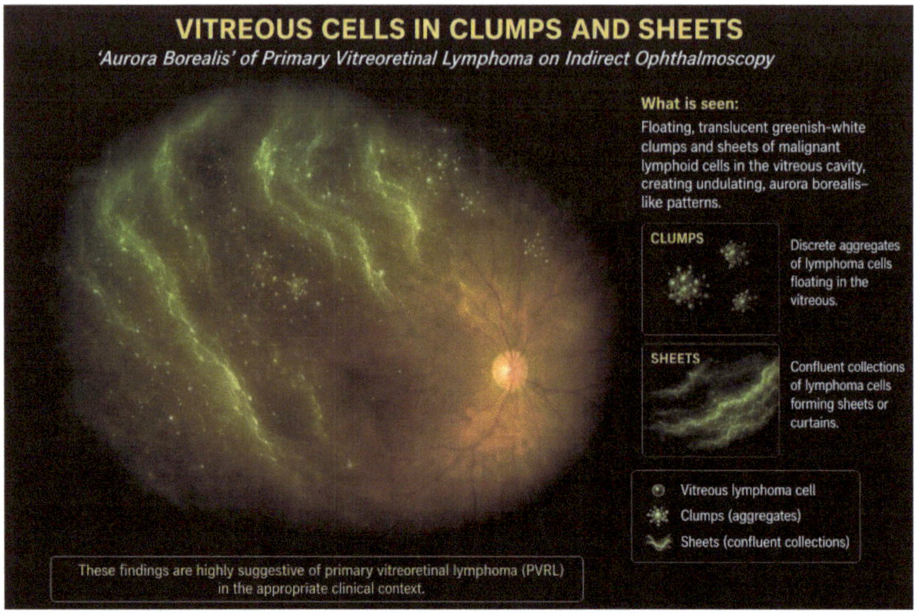

Figure 5.1 — Vitreous cells in clumps and sheets — the 'aurora borealis' of primary vitreoretinal lymphoma seen on indirect ophthalmoscopy.

5.2 Imaging signatures

SD-OCT in PVRL typically demonstrates hyper-reflective deposits in the sub-RPE or subretinal space, with disturbance of the ellipsoid zone and characteristic RPE undulations. As the disease progresses, larger nodular deposits may produce dome-shaped elevations. FAF reveals the granular 'leopard' pattern of alternating hyper- and hypo-autofluorescence — a sign often more diagnostic than colour fundus photography alone.[10,12] On FFA, the lesions may show blocked fluorescence or

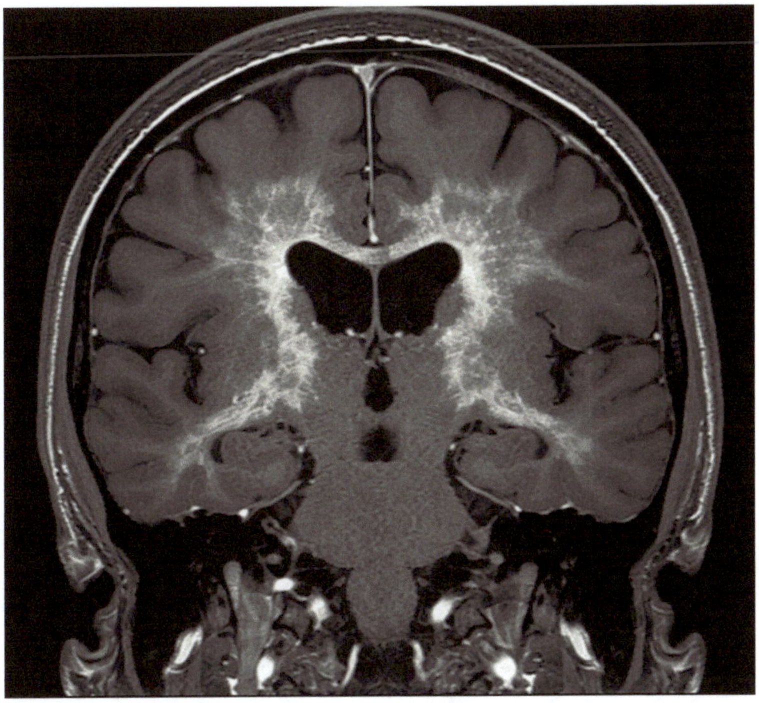

staining; on ICG, they typically appear as discrete hypofluorescent dark spots. MRI of the brain and orbits is mandatory and is the single most important systemic investigation.

Figure 5.2 — MRI brain coronal section showing periventricular enhancement in a patient with primary CNS lymphoma — the cerebral counterpart of the vitreoretinal disease.

TABLE 5.1

Diagnostic criteria of primary vitreoretinal lymphoma

Criterion	Detail
Cytology	Atypical lymphoid cells with high nuclear-to-cytoplasmic ratio, prominent nucleoli
Immunophenotype	CD20+, BCL-6+, MUM-1+, lambda or kappa restriction
Molecular	MYD88 L265P somatic mutation in ~70-90% of cases
Cytokines	Vitreous IL-10:IL-6 ratio >1 (sensitivity ~75%)

Imaging	OCT: sub-RPE deposits; FAF: granular pattern; MRI: CNS lesions

5.3 Diagnostic vitrectomy and molecular confirmation

Diagnostic vitrectomy remains the gold standard. The sample is examined for atypical lymphoid cells with high nuclear-to-cytoplasmic ratio, prominent nucleoli and frequent mitoses.[8,13] Immunophenotyping by flow cytometry demonstrates monoclonal B-cell populations (CD20+, CD19+, kappa or lambda light-chain restriction). The IL-10:IL-6 ratio greater than 1.0 supports the diagnosis with approximately 75% sensitivity.[9] The MYD88 L265P somatic mutation is identified in 70-90% of cases and now represents the most powerful single molecular marker, especially when cytological material is scant.[10]

A single non-diagnostic biopsy does not exclude PVRL. Repeat vitrectomy is indicated when suspicion remains and the first sample fails. CSF cytology and flow cytometry should be obtained in every confirmed case to complete the neurological staging.

FLOWCHART 5.1

Diagnostic and treatment pathway for primary vitreoretinal lymphoma

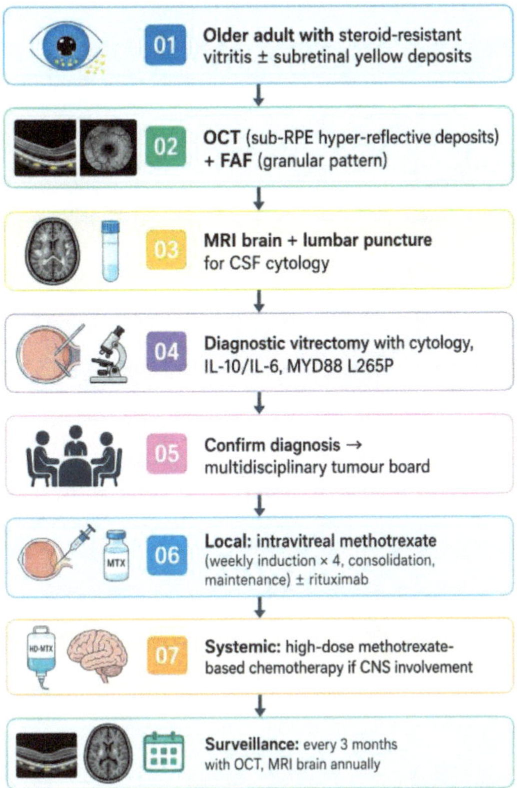

5.4 Treatment principles

Treatment of PVRL is multidisciplinary. Local control is achieved with intravitreal methotrexate 400 μg, typically delivered as weekly induction injections for four weeks, followed by twice-weekly consolidation and a monthly maintenance schedule. Intravitreal rituximab is an alternative or adjunctive option, particularly for steroid-sensitive disease.[15] When CNS involvement is documented or strongly suspected, systemic high-dose methotrexate-based chemotherapy is initiated under haemato-oncological supervision. The CALGB 50202 trial and subsequent series have established that combination therapy improves both survival and CNS relapse rates.[14]

Surveillance is lifelong. Patients are reviewed every three months with complete eye examination, OCT and FAF; MRI of the brain is repeated annually even after complete remission. Five-year survival, when treatment is initiated promptly, is now between 60% and 80% in most modern series.

CLINICAL PEARLS

- Suspect PVRL in any adult over 60 with bilateral, asymmetric, steroid-resistant vitritis.
- OCT and FAF are often diagnostic before cytology: look for sub-RPE deposits and 'leopard spotting'.
- MYD88 L265P is the most useful single molecular marker; test for it on every vitreous sample.
- Hold systemic steroids before diagnostic vitrectomy where clinically safe.

KEY POINTS

- PVRL and PCNSL form a continuum; CNS involvement develops in the majority of patients.
- Diagnosis combines clinical phenotype, OCT/FAF imaging, vitreous cytology, IL-10:IL-6 and MYD88.
- Therapy is intravitreal methotrexate (or rituximab) with systemic chemotherapy for CNS disease.
- Lifelong surveillance with OCT and annual MRI is essential.

SECTION II · CHAPTER 06

Metastatic Tumors and Paraneoplastic Syndromes

When the Eye Carries the Memory of Distant Disease

The eye is not an isolated organ. The choroid receives more blood flow per gram than almost any other tissue in the body, and that vascular generosity makes it a frequent destination for haematogenous metastasis. Choroidal metastasis is the most common intraocular malignancy in adults overall, even when uveal melanoma is included in the count. The list of primary tumours is led...

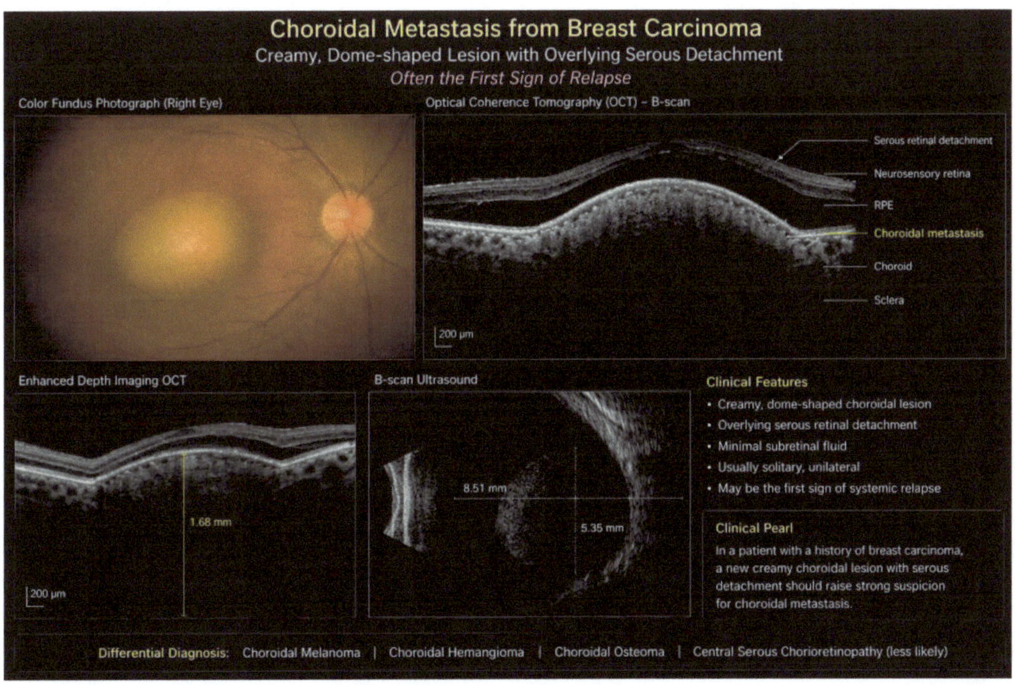

Figure 6.1 — Choroidal metastasis from breast carcinoma: a creamy, dome-shaped lesion with overlying serous detachment. Often the first sign of relapse.

CHAPTER 06

Metastatic Tumors and Paraneoplastic Syndromes

When the Eye Carries the Memory of Distant Disease

The eye is not an isolated organ. The choroid receives more blood flow per gram than almost any other tissue in the body, and that vascular generosity makes it a frequent destination for haematogenous metastasis. Choroidal metastasis is the most common intraocular malignancy in adults overall, even when uveal melanoma is included in the count. The list of primary tumours is led by breast (in women) and lung (in men), but any solid malignancy can metastasise to the eye. Beyond metastasis, paraneoplastic retinopathies — CAR, MAR — produce visual loss with minimal anterior segment signs and are often diagnosed only when systemic disease declares itself.[16,17,76]

6.1 Choroidal metastasis: the most common ocular tumour you will see

The clinical phenotype of choroidal metastasis is a creamy, dome-shaped or plateau-shaped subretinal lesion, often with overlying serous detachment. In contrast to uveal melanoma, metastatic lesions tend to be pale or yellow rather than pigmented, may be multifocal, and may be bilateral. Onset of symptoms is usually rapid — over weeks rather than months — and visual acuity reduction is often disproportionate to the lesion's apparent size because of the secondary retinal detachment.[17] B-scan ultrasound demonstrates a moderately reflective lesion with low to moderate internal reflectivity; OCT shows the dome elevation and subretinal fluid; ICG often reveals a hypofluorescent mass.

Choroidal metastasis is, in 20-30% of cases, the presenting feature of the systemic malignancy itself. This is why a careful systemic history — particularly for breast lumps, smoking history, weight loss, persistent cough or anaemia — is essential when faced with any new, atypical subretinal lesion in an adult. Where suspicion is high, urgent oncology referral for staging is the priority and may precede definitive ocular treatment.

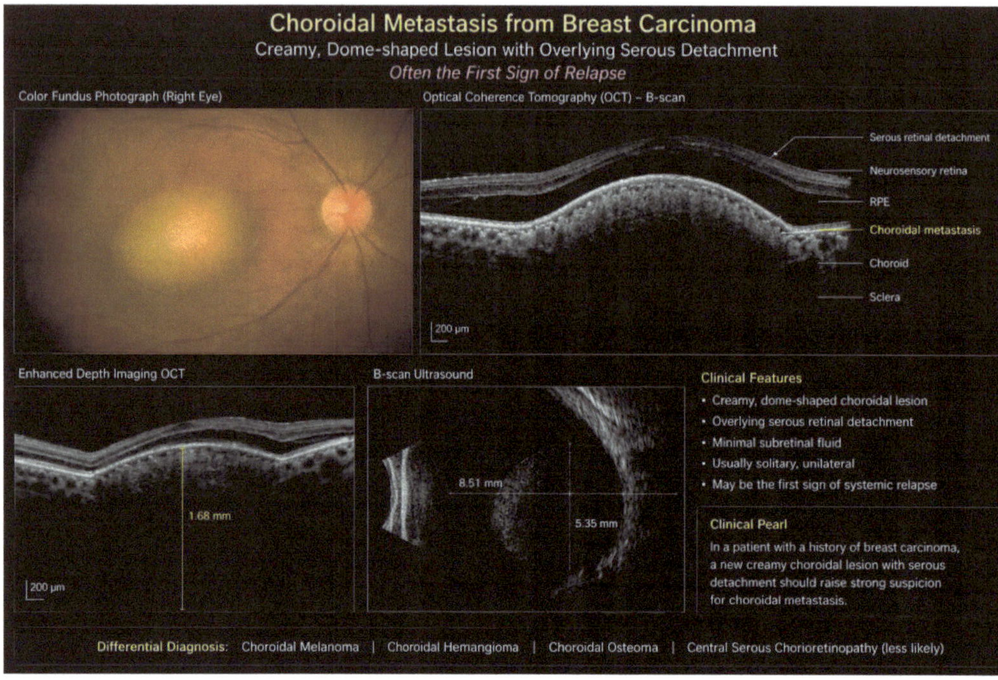

Figure 6.1 — Choroidal metastasis from breast carcinoma: a creamy, dome-shaped lesion with overlying serous detachment. Often the first sign of relapse.

6.2 Treatment of choroidal metastasis

Therapy is multidisciplinary. Systemic chemotherapy or targeted therapy directed at the primary malignancy usually has good ocular response — many breast and lung metastases regress with appropriate systemic treatment. External beam radiotherapy (20-30 Gy in 10-15 fractions) achieves local control in over 80% of cases. Stereotactic and proton beam radiotherapy are alternatives. Intravitreal anti-VEGF therapy is useful as an adjunct for secondary serous detachment.[17,75] Photodynamic therapy is occasionally used for small juxtafoveal lesions. Enucleation is reserved for blind, painful eyes.

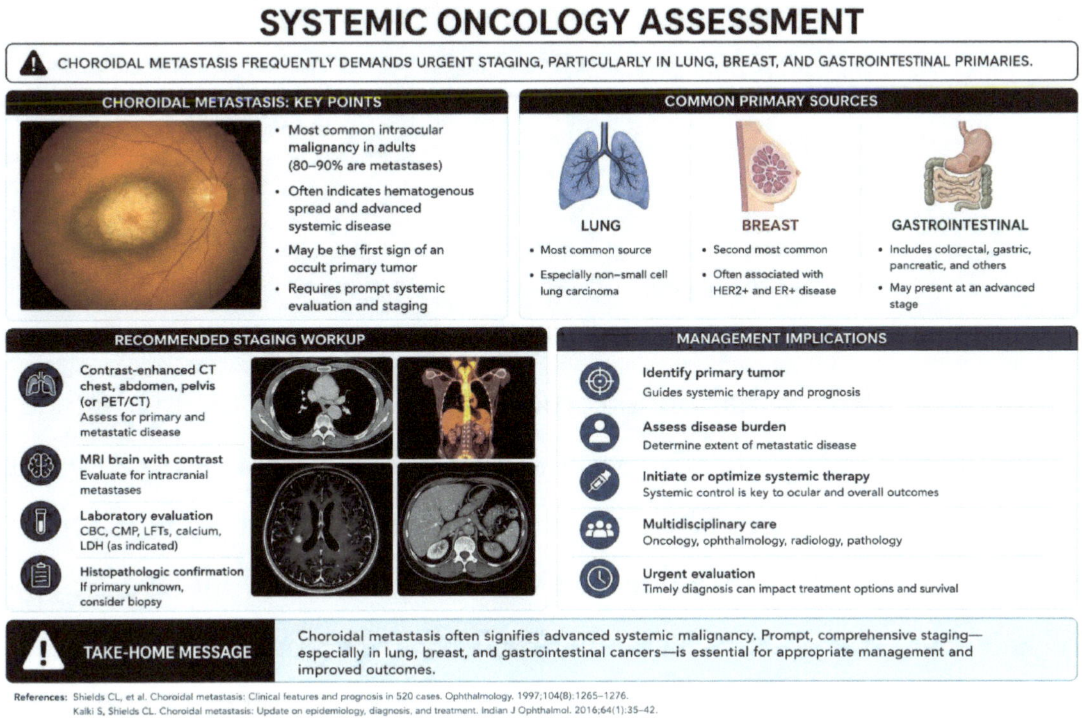

Figure 6.2 — Systemic oncology assessment. Choroidal metastasis frequently demands urgent staging, particularly in lung, breast, and gastrointestinal primaries.

6.3 Paraneoplastic retinopathies

Cancer-associated retinopathy (CAR), melanoma-associated retinopathy (MAR) and the related paraneoplastic optic neuritides are autoimmune syndromes in which antibodies generated against tumour antigens cross-react with retinal proteins. Patients present with progressive visual loss, photopsia, ring scotomas and dyschromatopsia. Anterior and posterior segment examination is often unremarkable; the diagnostic clue is the disproportion between symptoms and signs. Electroretinography is key — CAR produces a non-recordable or markedly attenuated ERG, MAR produces a characteristic negative ERG with normal a-wave and reduced b-wave.[76] Anti-recoverin (CAR) and anti-bipolar antibodies (MAR) can be tested in serum where available. Treatment is supportive and directed at the underlying malignancy; systemic immunosuppression has variable benefit.

6.4 Leukaemic and lymphomatous infiltration

Acute lymphoblastic leukaemia, acute myeloid leukaemia and the high-grade non-Hodgkin lymphomas may all involve the eye. Ocular leukaemia presents as pseudohypopyon, retinal haemorrhages with white centres (Roth spots), vitritis, and rarely an optic nerve infiltrate. In children with relapsed ALL, the eye may be the sanctuary site that announces the relapse weeks before the bone marrow does.[48,49,50] CBC, peripheral smear, LDH and bone-marrow review are essential when leukaemic infiltration is suspected; intraocular biopsy is reserved for atypical or refractory cases.

CLINICAL PEARLS

- Choroidal metastasis is the most common intraocular malignancy overall — always exclude in adult-onset, atypical subretinal lesions.
- Breast (women) and lung (men) are the commonest primaries.
- ERG is essential for paraneoplastic retinopathy diagnosis; antibodies confirm.
- Roth spots, pseudohypopyon and retinal infiltrates may herald systemic leukaemia.

KEY POINTS

- Choroidal metastasis may present before the primary tumour is known.
- Treatment combines oncological systemic therapy with EBRT for local control.
- Paraneoplastic retinopathies are diagnosed by symptom-sign mismatch and ERG.
- Haematological malignancies must be screened with peripheral smear in atypical uveitis.

SECTION II · CHAPTER 07

Uveal and Iris Tumors Mimicking Inflammation

Pigment, Posture, and the Iris That Bleeds Quietly

Uveal and iris tumours are particularly skilled masqueraders because the costume they wear — inflammation, pigment dispersion, raised intraocular pressure — is the same costume that benign disease wears. Diffuse iris melanoma may be diagnosed for years as 'pigment dispersion glaucoma'. A small choroidal melanoma may be treated as 'recurrent posterior uveitis'. Iridociliary cyst…

CHAPTER 07

Uveal and Iris Tumors Mimicking Inflammation

Pigment, Posture, and the Iris That Bleeds Quietly

Uveal and iris tumours are particularly skilled masqueraders because the costume they wear — inflammation, pigment dispersion, raised intraocular pressure — is the same costume that benign disease wears. Diffuse iris melanoma may be diagnosed for years as 'pigment dispersion glaucoma'. A small choroidal melanoma may be treated as 'recurrent posterior uveitis'. Iridociliary cysts may mimic chronic anterior uveitis. The remedy is the same in every case: careful documentation, high-frequency ultrasound biomicroscopy, and a willingness to refer early.[19,20,77,78]

7.1 Diffuse iris melanoma

Diffuse iris melanoma is the masquerade that most often deceives an experienced clinician because its presenting features — heterochromia, pigment dispersion, raised IOP, and even pseudohypopyon — are common in non-neoplastic disease. The clinical clue is asymmetric, progressive darkening of one iris in an adult, often associated with sentinel vessels and a stubbornly elevated intraocular pressure.[20] High-frequency UBM demonstrates a diffuse thickening of the iris stroma with infiltration of the angle. Where suspicion is high, fine-needle aspiration biopsy under experienced hands can establish the diagnosis. Treatment is enucleation in advanced cases, with proton beam radiotherapy reserved for selected smaller lesions.

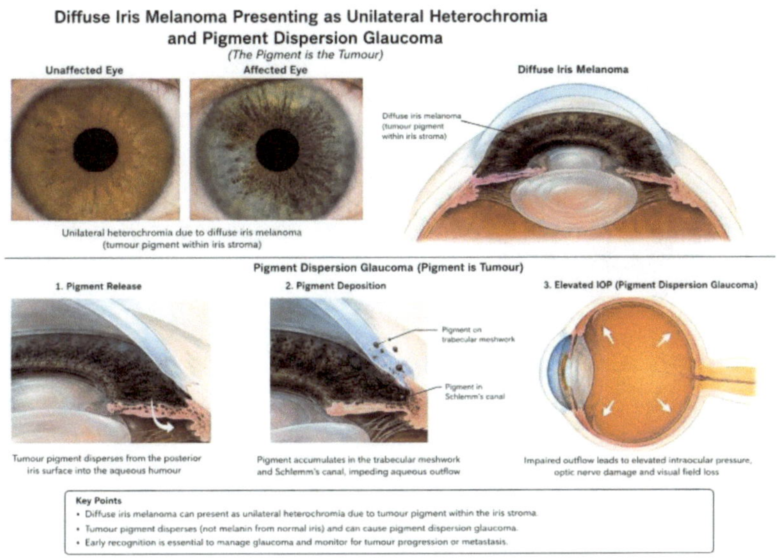

Figure 7.1 — Diffuse iris melanoma presenting as unilateral heterochromia and 'pigment dispersion glaucoma'. The pigment was the tumour.

7.2 Ring melanoma and ciliary body tumours

Ring melanoma of the ciliary body is a rare but classic masquerade. It presents as unilateral sentinel vessels, raised IOP, and an apparently isolated cataract — but careful gonioscopy reveals subtle angle pigmentation or anterior synechia, and high-frequency UBM uncovers a circumferential tumour. The lesion is often advanced at diagnosis because the costume of an 'asymmetric cataract' is so convincing.

7.3 Iridociliary cysts and pigmentary glaucoma

Iridociliary cysts are not malignant, but they masquerade as chronic anterior uveitis often enough to deserve their place in this chapter. They cause asymmetric pigment dispersion, focally raised IOP, and intermittent cells in the anterior chamber that respond only partially to topical steroids. High-frequency UBM is diagnostic and may obviate years of unnecessary therapy.[78] When cysts compress the trabecular meshwork and produce angle-closure, laser cystotomy or surgical excision is indicated.

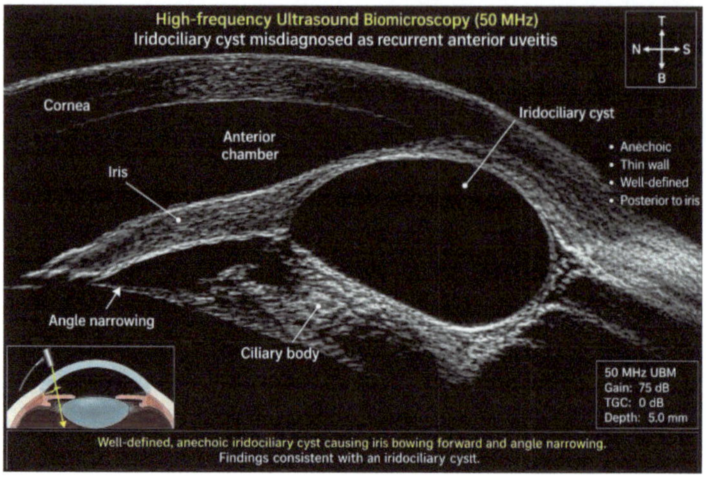

Figure 7.2 — High-frequency ultrasound biomicroscopy of an iridociliary cyst that had been treated for two years as recurrent anterior uveitis.

7.4 Choroidal melanoma mimicking posterior uveitis

Choroidal melanoma typically presents as a pigmented dome-shaped or mushroom-shaped lesion. But a small, amelanotic melanoma may be mistaken for a granuloma, an inflammatory infiltrate, or even a metastasis. The TFSOM-DIM mnemonic (Thickness >2 mm, subretinal Fluid, Symptoms, Orange pigment, Margin near optic disc, Diameter, Internal reflectivity, Mushroom shape) remains a useful predictor of malignancy in any suspicious choroidal lesion.[19] OCT, autofluorescence, B-scan and fluorescein angiography are complementary; referral to an ocular oncology centre is appropriate where doubt remains.

CLINICAL PEARLS

- Asymmetric heterochromia, sentinel vessels and a stubborn IOP in one eye are a triad to take seriously.
- High-frequency UBM uncovers iridociliary cysts and ring melanomas that the slit lamp misses.
- The TFSOM-DIM mnemonic helps grade the suspicion of any choroidal lesion.
- Refer to an ocular oncology centre when doubt remains — early referral preserves both eye and life.

KEY POINTS

- Diffuse iris melanoma is the most often-missed iris tumour because it imitates pigment dispersion.
- Ring melanoma may present as an asymmetric cataract.
- Iridociliary cysts are benign but a frequent masquerade of chronic anterior uveitis.
- Amelanotic choroidal melanoma can imitate granuloma or metastasis — TFSOM-DIM and B-scan distinguish.

SECTION II · CHAPTER 08

Ocular Surface Neoplasia and Paediatric Tumors

From the Conjunctival Edge to the Child's Retina

Ocular surface neoplasia and paediatric tumours sit at the bookends of the masquerade ball. Ocular surface squamous neoplasia (OSSN), conjunctival lymphoma and sebaceous gland carcinoma each imitate chronic surface inflammation. In children, retinoblastoma — particularly the diffuse infiltrating variant — can present as uveitis, pseudohypopyon or vitritis in older children, som…

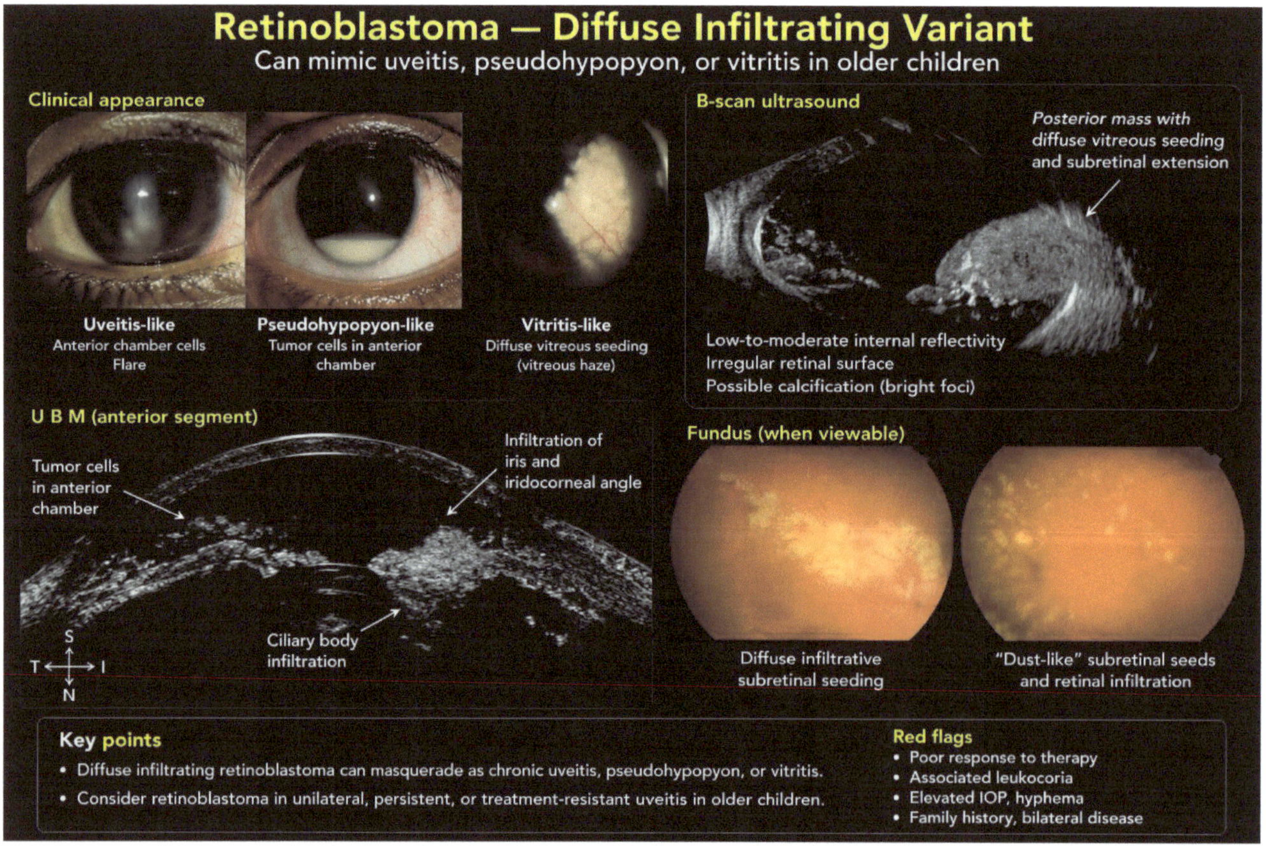

CHAPTER 08

Ocular Surface Neoplasia and Paediatric Tumors

From the Conjunctival Edge to the Child's Retina

Ocular surface neoplasia and paediatric tumours sit at the bookends of the masquerade ball. Ocular surface squamous neoplasia (OSSN), conjunctival lymphoma and sebaceous gland carcinoma each imitate chronic surface inflammation. In children, retinoblastoma — particularly the diffuse infiltrating variant — can present as uveitis, pseudohypopyon or vitritis in older children, sometimes leading to catastrophic delays in diagnosis. The cost of failure is high; the rewards of vigilance, exceptional.[21,22,23,24,47]

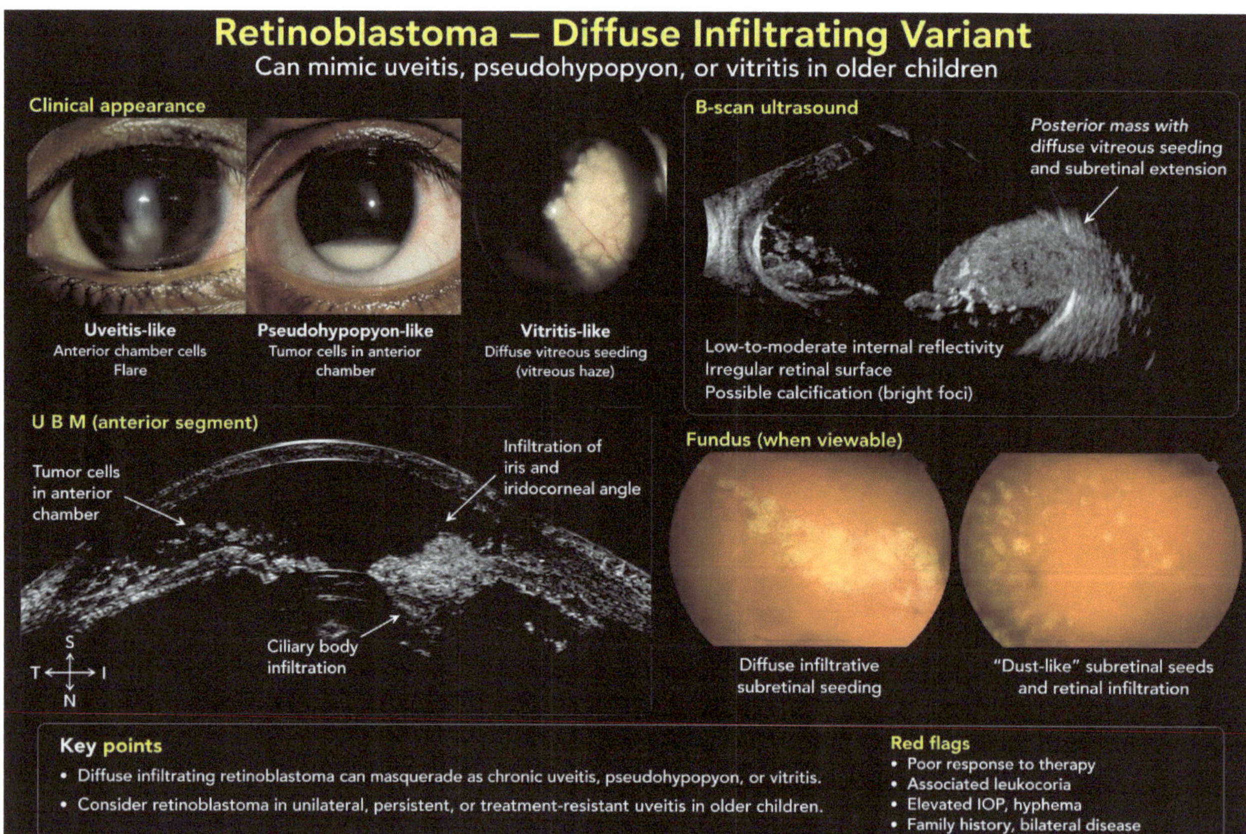

8.1 Ocular surface squamous neoplasia

OSSN typically presents as a unilateral, gelatinous, vascularised plaque with leukoplakic features at the limbus. It may have been treated for years as 'chronic conjunctivitis' or 'limbitis'. Diagnosis is clinical, supported by impression cytology and confirmed by excisional biopsy with histopathology. OCT of the anterior segment is increasingly used to demonstrate the characteristic thickened, hyperreflective epithelial layer with a sharp transition to normal epithelium. Treatment is excision with cryotherapy of the margins; topical mitomycin C, 5-fluorouracil or interferon-α2b are increasingly used as primary or adjuvant therapy.[22,23]

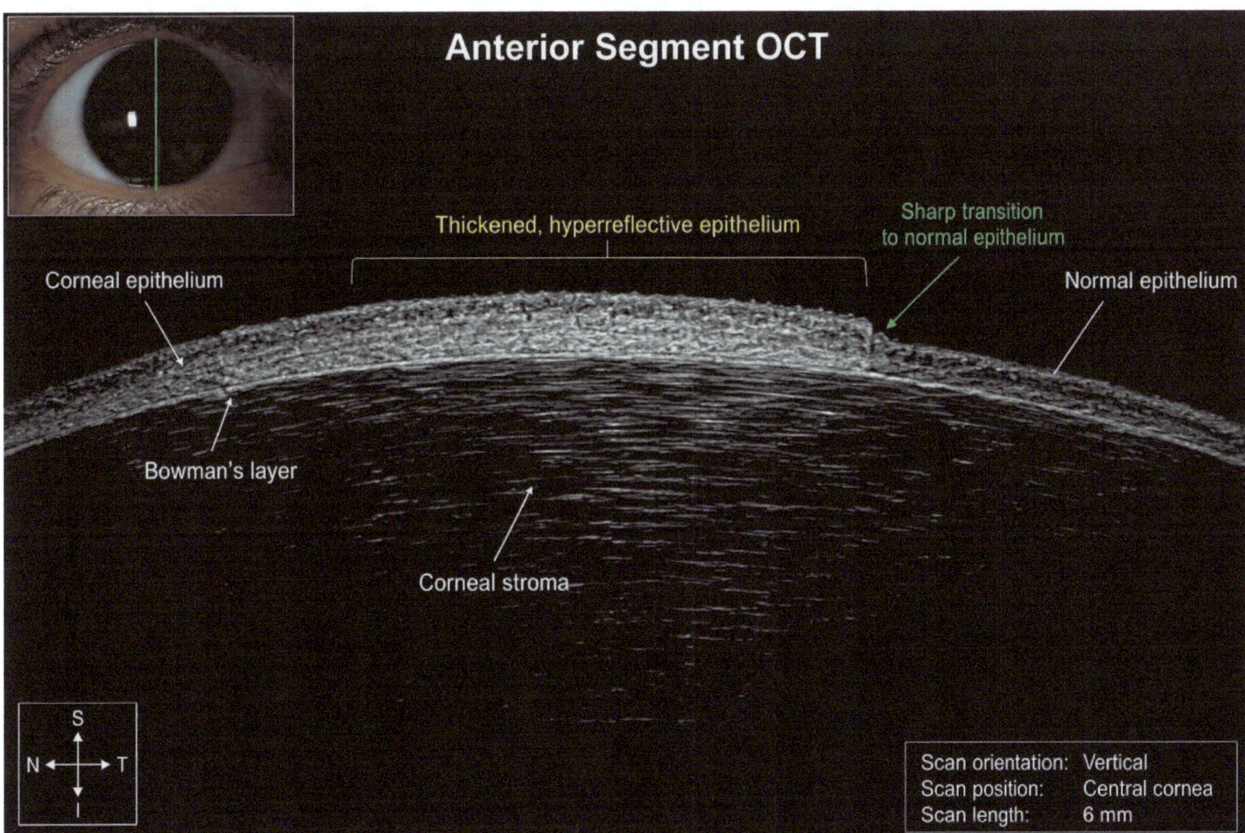

[Figure-8.1]-OCT of the anterior segment is increasingly used to demonstrate the characteristic thickened, hyperreflective epithelial layer with a sharp transition to normal epithelium.

8.2 Conjunctival lymphoma and conjunctival melanoma

Conjunctival lymphoma presents as a salmon-pink, smooth, fleshy subconjunctival infiltrate, most commonly in the fornix or bulbar conjunctiva. It may be misdiagnosed as a 'chronic episcleritis' or 'allergic conjunctivitis'. Most are extranodal marginal zone B-cell lymphomas (MALT type) but more aggressive subtypes occur.[22] Histopathology with immunophenotyping is diagnostic; treatment is low-dose external beam radiotherapy for localised disease and systemic therapy for diffuse or systemic involvement.

Conjunctival melanoma may arise de novo or, more commonly, from primary acquired melanosis with atypia (PAM). Pigmentation may be subtle or absent (amelanotic melanoma). Wide excision, cryotherapy and topical mitomycin C are the mainstays of therapy; sentinel lymph node biopsy is performed in high-risk cases.

8.3 Sebaceous gland carcinoma — the lethal mimic

Sebaceous gland carcinoma of the eyelid is the most lethal of the eyelid masquerades because it imitates chronic blepharitis, recurrent chalazion, or unilateral chronic conjunctivitis.[21] Any unilateral recalcitrant chalazion, particularly with associated madarosis, eyelid distortion or diffuse conjunctival redness, requires full-thickness biopsy including lid margin and conjunctiva. Map biopsies of the conjunctiva may be needed to detect pagetoid spread. Treatment is wide excision with frozen-section control; mortality from regional and distant metastasis remains 10-30% in advanced cases.

8.4 Paediatric tumours: retinoblastoma masquerading as uveitis

Retinoblastoma in children under three almost always presents with leucocoria or strabismus. In children between three and seven, however, the diffuse infiltrating variant may present as 'unilateral chronic uveitis' with pseudohypopyon and vitritis. The eye may have been treated with topical and periocular steroids for months before the diagnosis is made.[24,47] Examination under anaesthesia with detailed indirect ophthalmoscopy, B-scan ultrasound (looking for calcification), and MRI are the diagnostic tools of choice. Vitreous biopsy is contraindicated because of the risk of extraocular tumour spread; if performed in exceptional circumstances, it must be done with extreme care and specialised technique.

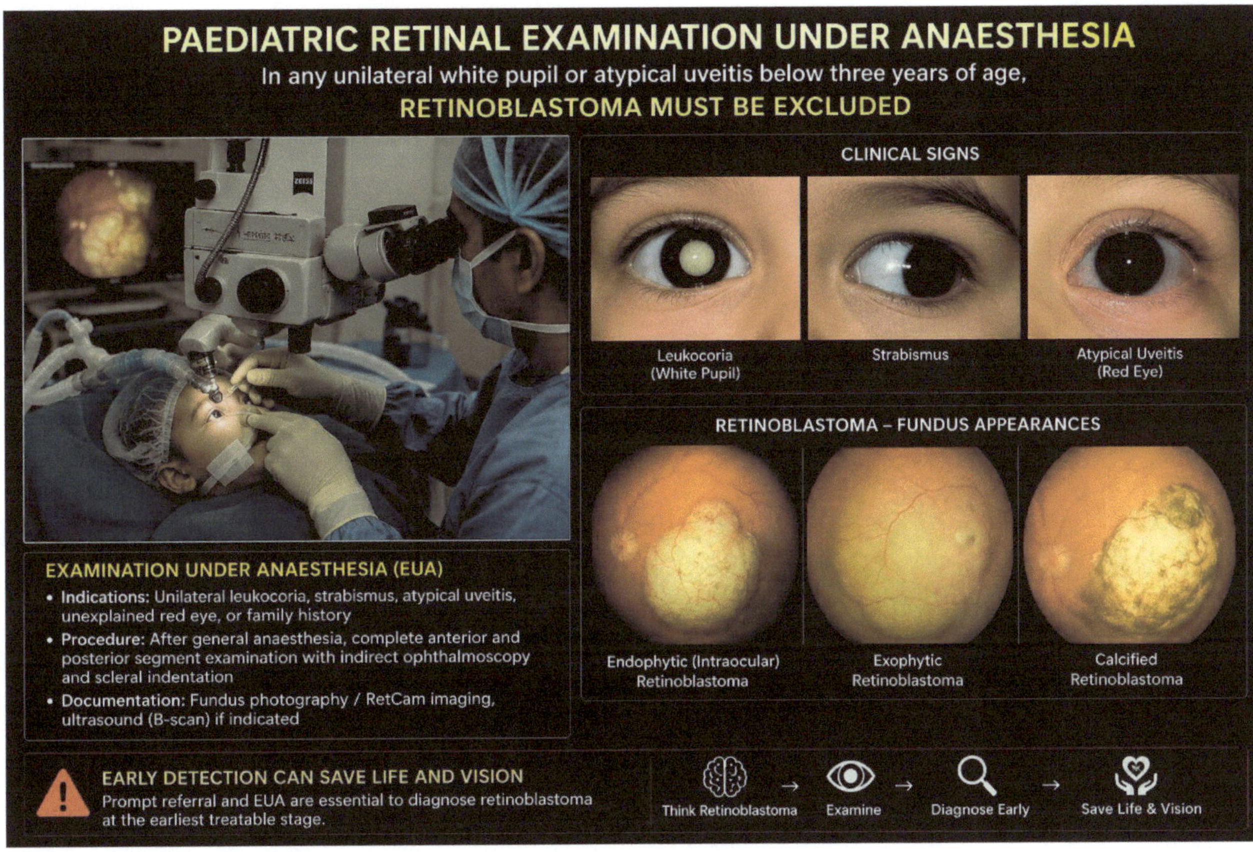

Figure 8.2 — Paediatric retinal examination under anaesthesia. In any unilateral white pupil or atypical uveitis below three years of age, retinoblastoma must be excluded.

CLINICAL PEARLS

- Any unilateral recalcitrant chalazion with madarosis is sebaceous gland carcinoma until biopsy says otherwise.
- Salmon-pink subconjunctival infiltrates are MALT lymphoma until proven otherwise.
- OSSN is increasingly treated topically — but biopsy or impression cytology first.
- Children with apparent uveitis under three years need retinoblastoma exclusion before any steroid escalation; the diffuse infiltrating variant may present older with pseudohypopyon.

KEY POINTS

- Eyelid and conjunctival neoplasms are 'surface masquerades' of inflammation.
- Wide excision with histological margin control is the foundation of surgical management.
- Topical chemotherapeutic agents (MMC, 5-FU, interferon) have transformed OSSN management.
- Retinoblastoma in older children may present as uveitis — never biopsy a suspected retinoblastoma vitreously.

SECTION III

Non-Neoplastic Masquerades

Infections that imitate sterile inflammation, autoimmunity that mimics infection, drugs that whisper the language of uveitis, and the rare paediatric entities that every clinician should learn to suspect early.

SECTION III · CHAPTER 09

Infectious Masquerades

Pathogens in the Costume of Inflammation

Infectious masquerades sit at the boundary of two clinical disciplines and demand a comfortable command of both. They are the diseases that the eye doctor must learn to share with the infectious diseases physician — particularly ocular syphilis ('the new great imitator'), ocular tuberculosis, ocular toxoplasmosis with atypical

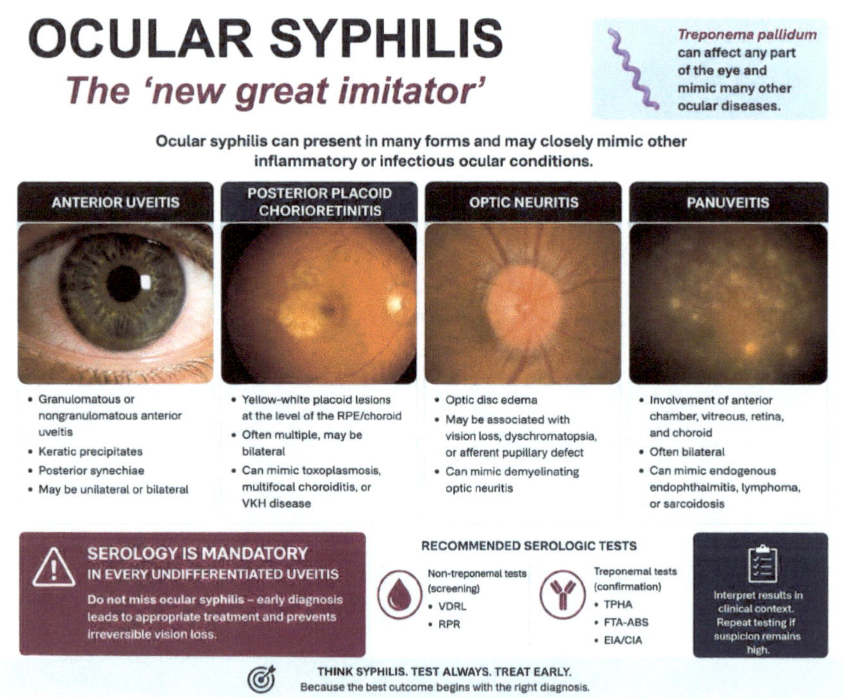

features, viral retinitides in the immunocompetent, ...

Figure 9.1 — Ocular syphilis, the 'new great imitator', can present as anterior uveitis, posterior placoid chorioretinitis, optic neuritis or panuveitis. Serology is mandatory in every undifferentiated uveitis.

CHAPTER 09

Infectious Masquerades

Pathogens in the Costume of Inflammation

Infectious masquerades sit at the boundary of two clinical disciplines and demand a comfortable command of both. They are the diseases that the eye doctor must learn to share with the infectious diseases physician — particularly ocular syphilis ('the new great imitator'), ocular tuberculosis, ocular toxoplasmosis with atypical features, viral retinitides in the immunocompetent, and the endogenous endophthalmitides that present as panuveitis. Each of them is curable. Each of them is missed when serology and systemic workup are deferred while topical steroids are escalated.[31,34,35,67]

9.1 Ocular syphilis — the new great imitator

Syphilis has been called 'the great imitator' since the time of Osler, and since 2010 its global incidence has risen sharply in both high- and low-income settings. Ocular syphilis may present at any stage of infection. The classical picture is acute syphilitic posterior placoid chorioretinitis — a yellow placoid lesion at the macula with retinal thickening — but ocular syphilis can present as anterior uveitis, intermediate uveitis, panuveitis, optic neuritis, retinal vasculitis or isolated scleritis.[34,35] The cardinal teaching is that every undifferentiated uveitis must have syphilis serology checked at first presentation; the cost is small, the consequences of missed diagnosis are large.

Diagnosis is by combination treponemal (FTA-ABS or TPHA) and non-treponemal (VDRL or RPR) serology; CSF examination is indicated where neurological involvement is suspected or where ocular signs are advanced. Treatment follows the protocols for neurosyphilis: intravenous benzylpenicillin 18-24 million units daily for 10-14 days, with public health notification. Visual recovery, when treatment is early, is often dramatic.

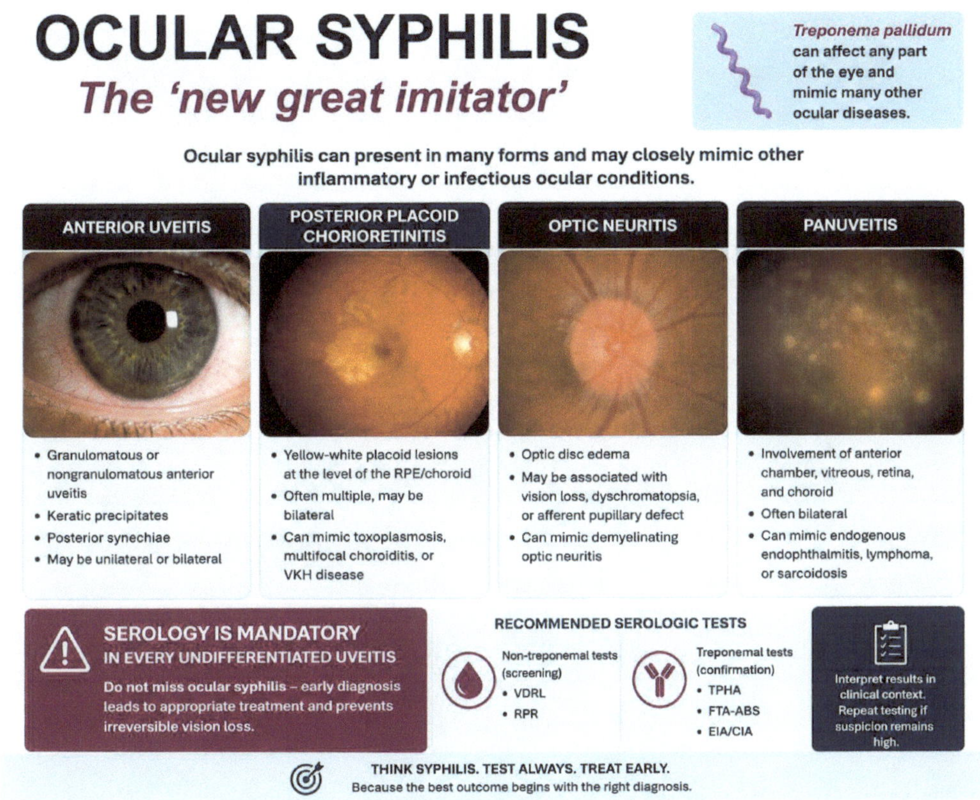

Figure 9.1 — Ocular syphilis, the 'new great imitator', can present as anterior uveitis, posterior placoid chorioretinitis, optic neuritis or panuveitis. Serology is mandatory in every undifferentiated uveitis.

TABLE 9.1

Tests indicated in every undifferentiated panuveitis (masquerade screen)

Test	Rationale
VDRL/RPR + FTA-ABS or TPHA	Syphilis serology — never omit
IGRA (QuantiFERON / T-SPOT)	Latent or active ocular tuberculosis
HIV serology	Risk of opportunistic infection / lymphoma
Chest imaging (X-ray ± HRCT)	Sarcoidosis, tuberculosis, malignancy
ACE, lysozyme	Sarcoidosis support
ANCA, ANA, dsDNA	Vasculitis, autoimmune connective tissue disease
CBC + peripheral smear + LDH	Haematologic malignancy, leukaemia

9.2 Ocular tuberculosis

Ocular tuberculosis is endemic in much of Asia, Africa and Latin America, and increasingly seen in returning travellers and migrants in the West. Phenotypes include serpiginous-like choroiditis (the classical TB-related phenotype), multifocal choroiditis, retinal vasculitis with neovascular complications (Eales-like disease), anterior granulomatous uveitis with iris nodules, and panuveitis.[31,32,42] The diagnostic difficulty is that M. tuberculosis is rarely cultured from the eye and that latent infection (positive IGRA) is common in endemic regions. The COTS-1 multicentre study demonstrated that anti-tubercular therapy with corticosteroids achieves good visual outcomes in selected cases and that the choice of patients for treatment depends on a combination of clinical phenotype, IGRA, chest imaging and response to a treatment trial.[32]

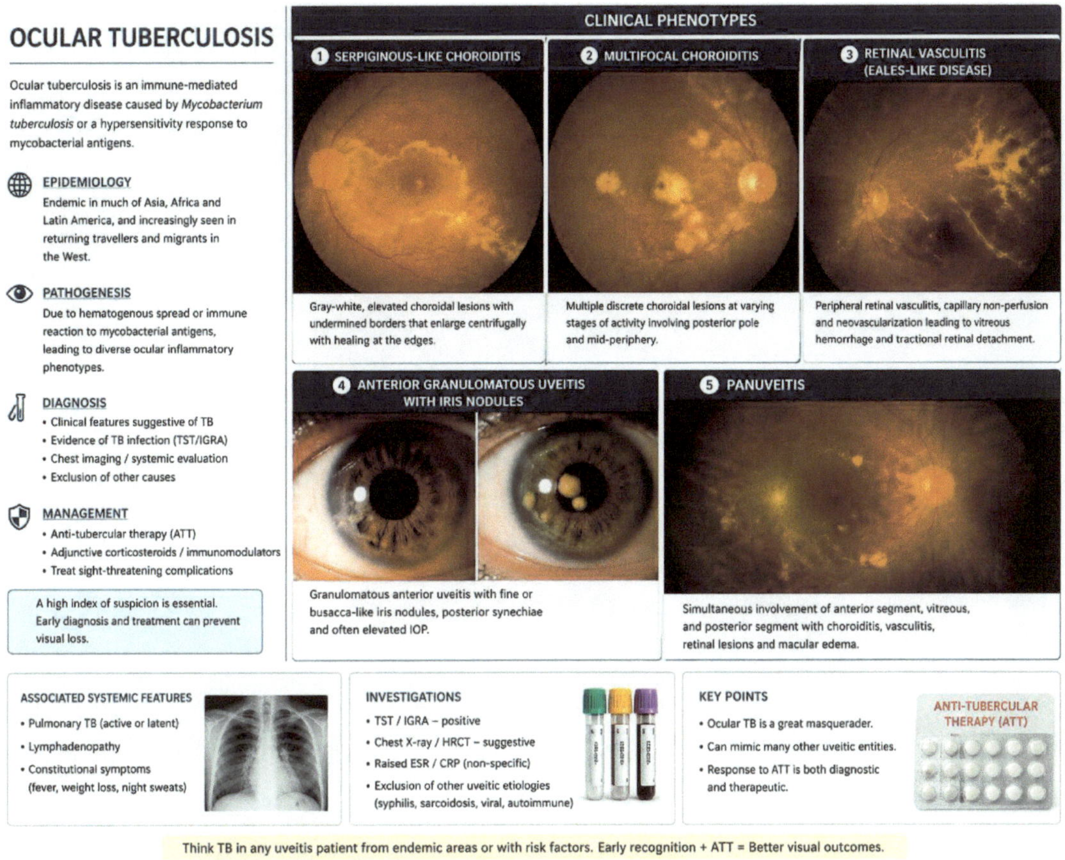

9.3 Viral retinitides and atypical toxoplasmosis

Acute retinal necrosis (ARN, classically VZV or HSV-1) and progressive outer retinal necrosis (PORN, VZV in profoundly immunocompromised patients) present as panuveitis with peripheral retinitis and may be misdiagnosed as 'severe posterior uveitis'. Cytomegalovirus retinitis in immunocompetent patients is increasingly recognised and may present as anterior uveitis with corneal endotheliitis ('Posner-Schlossman'-like phenotype) or as smouldering posterior pole disease. Diagnosis is by aqueous PCR. Treatment is intravitreal antiviral therapy (ganciclovir, foscarnet) with systemic backbone in immunocompromise.[44,58,73]

Toxoplasmosis is usually obvious — a focal area of retinochoroiditis adjacent to an old pigmented scar — but atypical phenotypes (punctate outer retinitis, neuroretinitis, retinal vasculitis, scleritis) occur, particularly in older or immunocompromised patients. Serology is rarely useful in endemic populations; aqueous PCR for T. gondii confirms the diagnosis.[33,57]

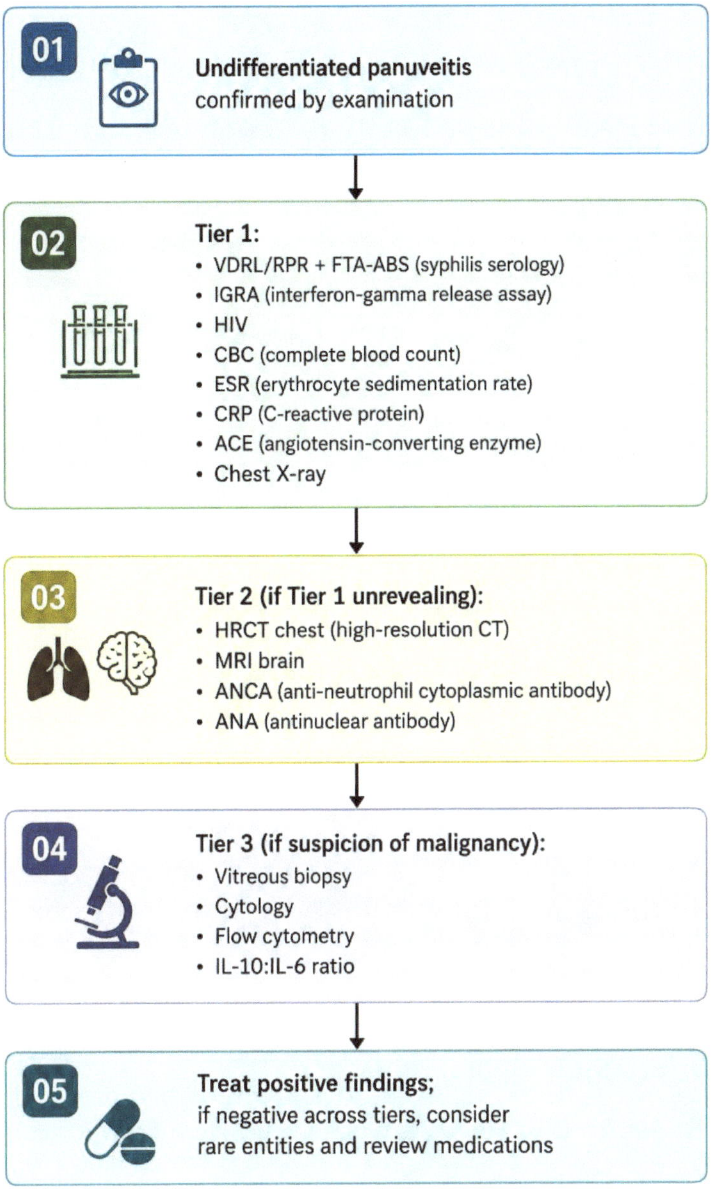

9.4 Endogenous endophthalmitis and Whipple disease

Endogenous endophthalmitis arises by haematogenous seeding of the eye from a systemic focus — often a urinary tract infection, an indwelling intravenous catheter, an infective endocarditis, or, in endemic regions, a hepatic abscess due to Klebsiella pneumoniae. The eye finding is a severe panuveitis with vitreous opacification and chorioretinitis; systemic illness is usually overt. Diagnosis is by vitreous tap with Gram stain, culture and broad-range PCR; treatment combines intravitreal antimicrobials with systemic therapy directed by blood cultures. Whipple disease

(Tropheryma whipplei) is a rare but well-described cause of chronic vitritis and retinitis with characteristic PAS-positive foamy macrophages; small bowel biopsy or aqueous/vitreous PCR is diagnostic.[59]

CLINICAL PEARLS

- Every uveitis without a clear diagnosis must have syphilis serology checked at first visit.
- Ocular syphilis responds dramatically to neurosyphilis-protocol intravenous penicillin.
- Ocular TB is diagnosed by clinical phenotype + IGRA + chest imaging + treatment response; the COTS studies guide therapy.
- Aqueous PCR for HSV/VZV/CMV/T. gondii is now standard care for atypical retinitis.

KEY POINTS

- Syphilis, TB, viral retinitides and endogenous endophthalmitis are 'curable masquerades' if diagnosed early.
- A standard tier-1 masquerade screen (syphilis, IGRA, HIV, chest imaging) belongs in every undifferentiated panuveitis.
- Aqueous PCR has transformed atypical anterior and posterior uveitis workup.
- Endogenous endophthalmitis often signals systemic illness — investigate the body, not just the eye.

SECTION III · CHAPTER 10

Autoimmune and Granulomatous Mimics

Self Against Self, Mimicking Foreign Invasion

Autoimmune and granulomatous disease is a master class in clinical mimicry. Sarcoidosis is responsible for some of the most beautifully reproducible imitations of every uveitis category. IgG4-related disease has emerged as a distinct entity in the last fifteen years and presents with orbital and lacrimal-gland enlargement, scleritis and uveitis. Granulomatosis with polyangiitis…

Figure 10.1 — High-resolution CT chest demonstrating bilateral hilar lymphadenopathy.
Ocular sarcoidosis often whispers from the chest before it shouts from the eye.

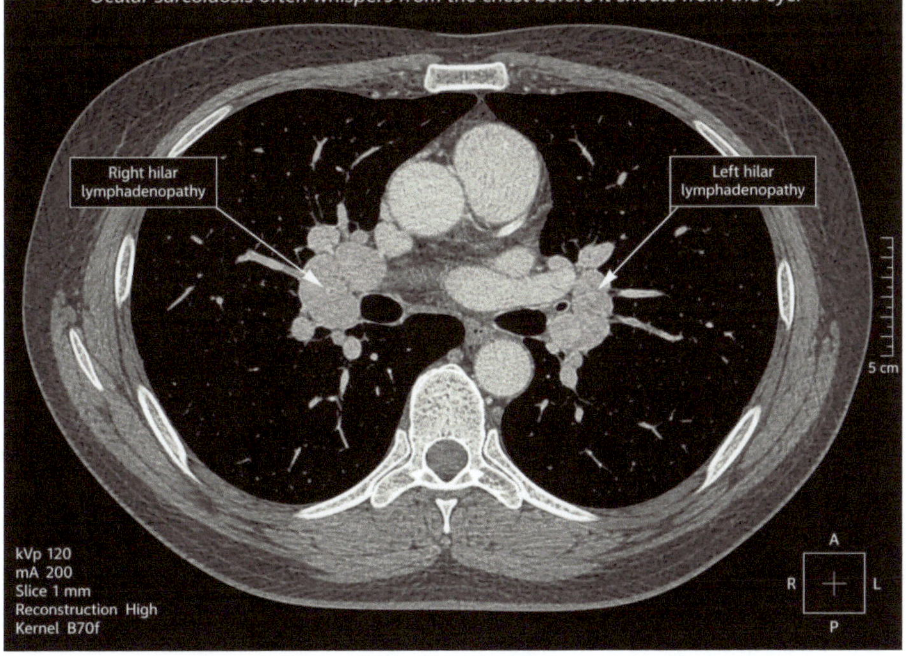

Figure 10.1 — High-resolution CT chest demonstrating bilateral hilar lymphadenopathy. Ocular sarcoidosis often whispers from the chest before it shouts from the eye.

CHAPTER 10

Autoimmune and Granulomatous Mimics

Self Against Self, Mimicking Foreign Invasion

Autoimmune and granulomatous disease is a master class in clinical mimicry. Sarcoidosis is responsible for some of the most beautifully reproducible imitations of every uveitis category. IgG4-related disease has emerged as a distinct entity in the last fifteen years and presents with orbital and lacrimal-gland enlargement, scleritis and uveitis. Granulomatosis with polyangiitis (GPA) imitates infectious scleritis, peripheral ulcerative keratitis and posterior scleritis. Each entity rewards the clinician who looks beyond the eye.[29,30,39,40,41,62,63,64]

10.1 Ocular sarcoidosis

Ocular sarcoidosis is the prototypical granulomatous masquerade. It can present at any age but classically affects two demographic peaks: women in their twenties to forties and a second peak in the seventh decade. Manifestations span the entire eye: dry eye and lacrimal gland enlargement, granulomatous anterior uveitis with mutton-fat keratic precipitates and iris nodules, intermediate uveitis with snowballs, posterior uveitis with candle-wax drippings and choroidal granulomas, optic nerve granulomas, and orbital involvement.[29,30] The 2019 International Workshop on Ocular Sarcoidosis revised criteria streamlined the diagnostic categories and are the practical reference for daily use.

Investigation in suspected ocular sarcoidosis includes chest radiograph and HRCT, serum ACE and lysozyme, calcium, and where systemic features are present, biopsy of the lacrimal gland, conjunctival nodules or transbronchial lung tissue. Treatment is systemic corticosteroids with steroid-sparing immunosuppression for chronic disease; biologic therapy (anti-TNF) is used in refractory or chronic cases.

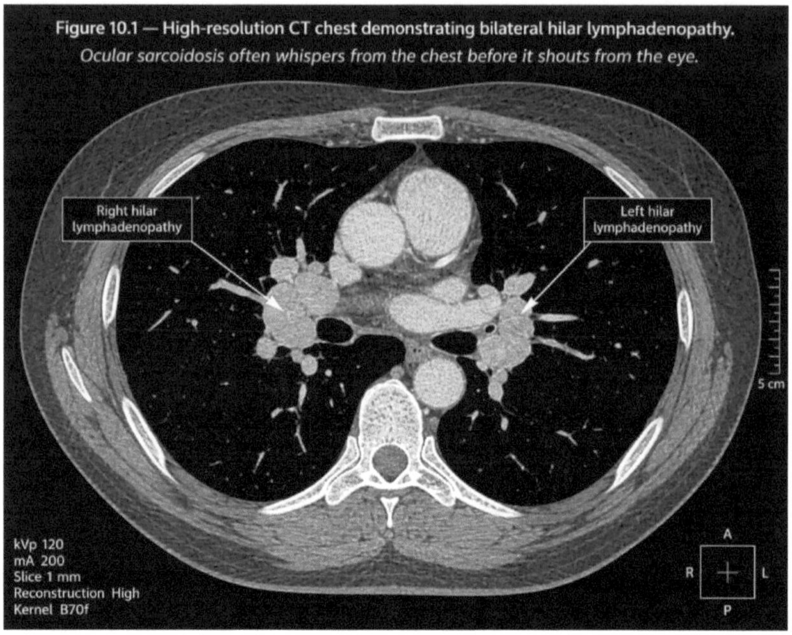

Figure 10.1 — High-resolution CT chest demonstrating bilateral hilar lymphadenopathy. Ocular sarcoidosis often whispers from the chest before it shouts from the eye.

10.2 IgG4-related ophthalmic disease

IgG4-related disease is now a recognised cause of bilateral lacrimal gland enlargement, orbital pseudotumour, scleritis and uveitis. Diagnostic criteria require histopathology showing dense IgG4-positive plasma cell infiltrate (>10 per high-power field or IgG4:IgG ratio >40%), storiform fibrosis and obliterative phlebitis. Serum IgG4 is elevated in about half of cases. Patients respond exceptionally well to corticosteroids, but relapse is common and rituximab is increasingly used as maintenance therapy.[39]

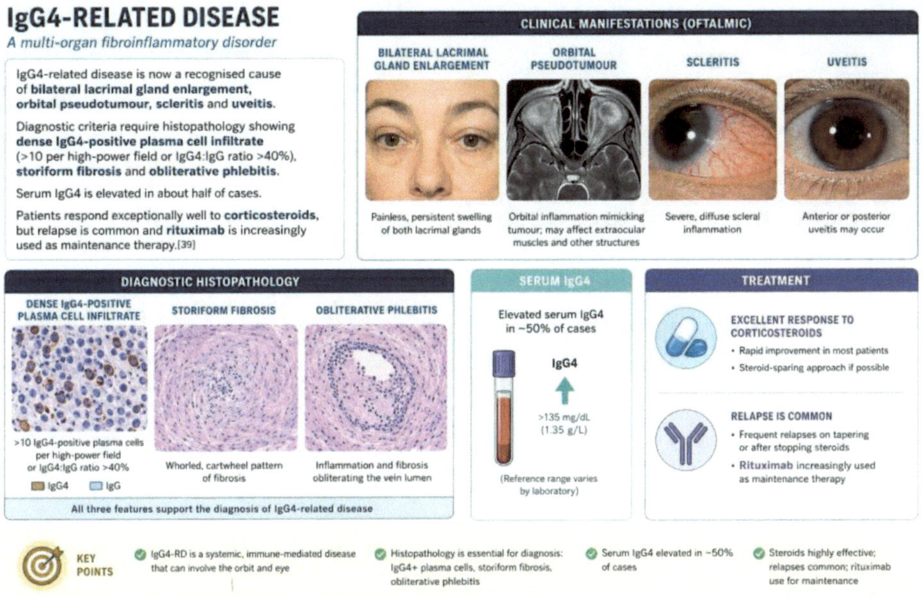

10.3 Granulomatosis with polyangiitis

Granulomatosis with polyangiitis presents with ocular involvement in 30-50% of cases. Manifestations include peripheral ulcerative keratitis, necrotising scleritis, retinal vasculitis, optic neuropathy and orbital pseudotumour with bony erosion.[40,41] The classical 'red eye that won't settle' — particularly with adjacent corneal melting — should always prompt anti-PR3 ANCA testing and urgent rheumatology consultation. Treatment combines high-dose corticosteroids with cyclophosphamide or rituximab; aggressive therapy is essential to prevent globe perforation and to protect renal and pulmonary function.

10.4 Vogt-Koyanagi-Harada and sympathetic ophthalmia

Vogt-Koyanagi-Harada (VKH) disease and sympathetic ophthalmia are not themselves masquerades, but they masquerade frequently as other panuveitides — particularly drug-induced (MEK inhibitor) serous retinopathies and choroidal metastasis with multiple bilateral foci. The characteristic features are bilateral exudative retinal detachments with thickened choroid on EDI-OCT, integumentary changes (poliosis, vitiligo) and neurological features in VKH; a history of penetrating ocular trauma or intraocular surgery in sympathetic ophthalmia.[80,83] Treatment is high-dose corticosteroids with prolonged taper, often with steroid-sparing immunosuppression.

CLINICAL PEARLS

- Sarcoid can imitate anterior, intermediate, posterior or panuveitis — always check chest imaging and ACE.
- Bilateral lacrimal gland enlargement with elevated serum IgG4 is IgG4-related disease until proven otherwise.
- Necrotising scleritis with peripheral ulcerative keratitis demands urgent ANCA testing.
- MEK inhibitors can imitate VKH — review the medication list before steroid escalation.

KEY POINTS

- Autoimmune masquerades typically declare themselves through extraocular features; the eye is only the door.
- Histopathology remains the gold standard for IgG4-related disease and sarcoidosis.
- ANCA testing is mandatory in necrotising scleritis or peripheral ulcerative keratitis.
- Steroid-sparing agents and biologics are the modern mainstay of refractory autoimmune ocular disease.

SECTION III · CHAPTER 11

Drug-Induced and Iatrogenic Masquerades

When Therapy Becomes the Disease

Drug-induced and iatrogenic masquerades are the masquerades the modern clinician most often manufactures unintentionally. The pharmacopoeia has expanded — bisphosphonates for osteoporosis, rifabutin for atypical mycobacteria,

MEK and BRAF inhibitors for melanoma, immune-checkpoint inhibitors across

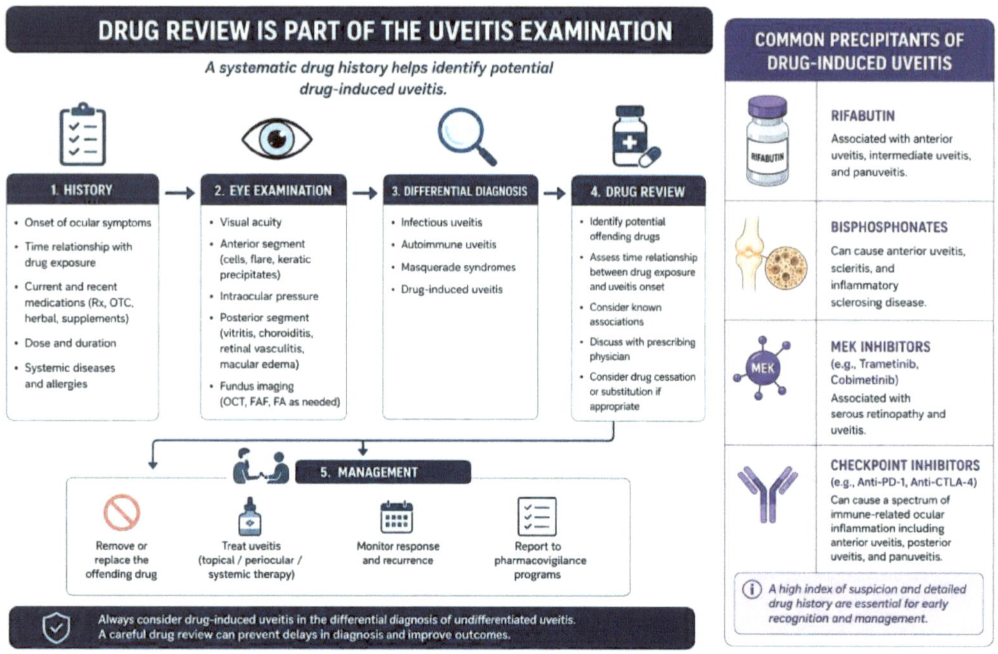

oncology — and each new class has brought a new pattern of ocular adverse effect…

Figure 11.1 — Drug review is part of the uveitis examination. Rifabutin, bisphosphonates, MEK and checkpoint inhibitors are common precipitants of drug-induced uveitis.

CHAPTER 11

Drug-Induced and Iatrogenic Masquerades

When Therapy Becomes the Disease

Drug-induced and iatrogenic masquerades are the masquerades the modern clinician most often manufactures unintentionally. The pharmacopoeia has expanded — bisphosphonates for osteoporosis, rifabutin for atypical mycobacteria, MEK and BRAF inhibitors for melanoma, immune-checkpoint inhibitors across oncology — and each new class has brought a new pattern of ocular adverse effects. Recognising drug-induced uveitis is often the difference between a one-week diagnosis and a one-year misadventure.[43]

11.1 Common offenders

Rifabutin, used in HIV and atypical mycobacterial infection, classically produces a bilateral hypopyon anterior uveitis. Bisphosphonates can cause anterior uveitis, scleritis or episcleritis, typically within days to weeks of the first infusion. Cidofovir, used for resistant CMV retinitis, causes anterior uveitis and hypotony. MEK inhibitors (trametinib, cobimetinib) produce serous retinal detachments that mimic VKH or central serous chorioretinopathy. BRAF inhibitors (vemurafenib, dabrafenib) cause anterior or panuveitis. Interferon-α produces a retinopathy with cotton wool spots and haemorrhages. Immune-checkpoint inhibitors (ipilimumab, nivolumab, pembrolizumab) induce a spectrum from anterior uveitis to VKH-like panuveitis with integumentary signs.[43] Table 11.1 collects the principal offenders for quick clinical reference.

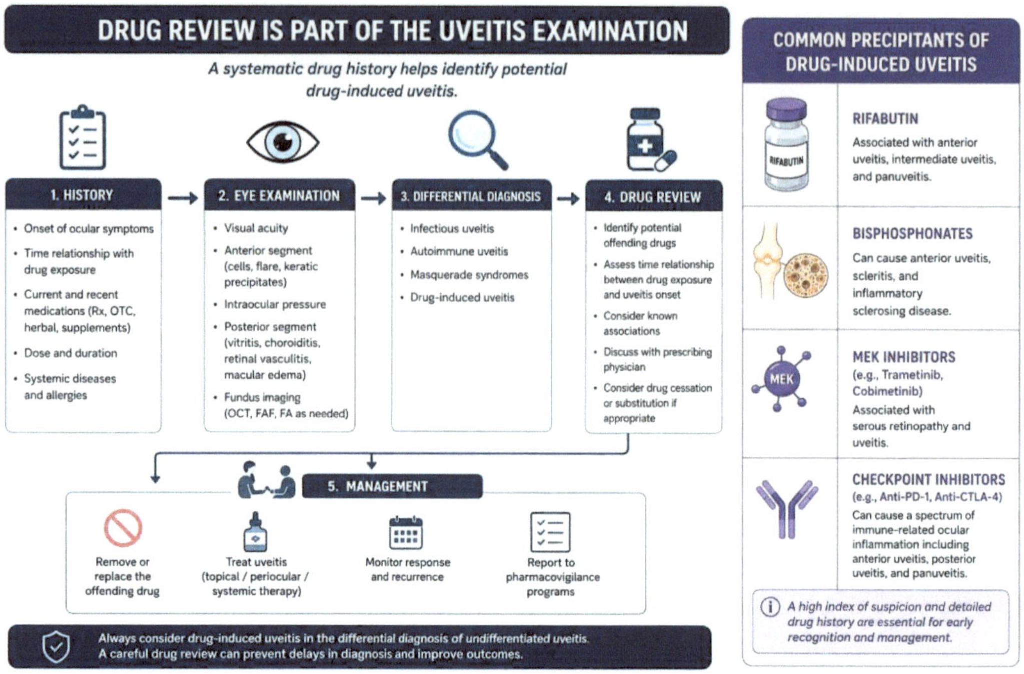

Figure 11.1 — Drug review is part of the uveitis examination. Rifabutin, bisphosphonates, MEK and checkpoint inhibitors are common precipitants of drug-induced uveitis.

TABLE 11.1

Common drug-induced ocular masquerades

Drug	Ocular Manifestation
Rifabutin	Hypopyon anterior uveitis, often bilateral
Bisphosphonates	Anterior uveitis, scleritis
Cidofovir	Anterior uveitis, hypotony
MEK inhibitors (trametinib)	Serous retinal detachments mimicking VKH or CSCR
BRAF inhibitors	Anterior uveitis, panuveitis
Checkpoint inhibitors (ipilimumab/nivolumab)	Uveitis, VKH-like syndrome, optic neuritis
Interferon-α	Retinopathy with cotton wool spots and haemorrhages

11.2 Recognising and managing drug-induced disease

The first step is suspicion: every uveitis history must include a complete medication review with attention to recently introduced drugs. The second is co-management: continuing or discontinuing the offending agent is rarely a unilateral ophthalmic decision, especially in oncology patients on life-prolonging therapy. The third is treatment: most drug-induced uveitides respond promptly to topical corticosteroids and cycloplegia, with systemic corticosteroids reserved for severe or bilateral disease. When the offending drug must be continued, a tailored steroid regimen with regular monitoring may be appropriate.

11.3 Iatrogenic masquerades: retained foreign bodies and silicone

Retained intraocular foreign bodies — particularly small metallic fragments after high-velocity trauma — may produce chronic anterior or panuveitis that fails to respond to steroids. Siderosis from retained iron and chalcosis from retained copper produce characteristic discolorations of the iris and lens with progressive retinal dysfunction. Ultrasound, CT and MRI (where the IOFB is non-ferrous) are the diagnostic tools.[78] Silicone oil tamponade after vitrectomy occasionally produces a chronic granulomatous uveitis that resolves with silicone removal.

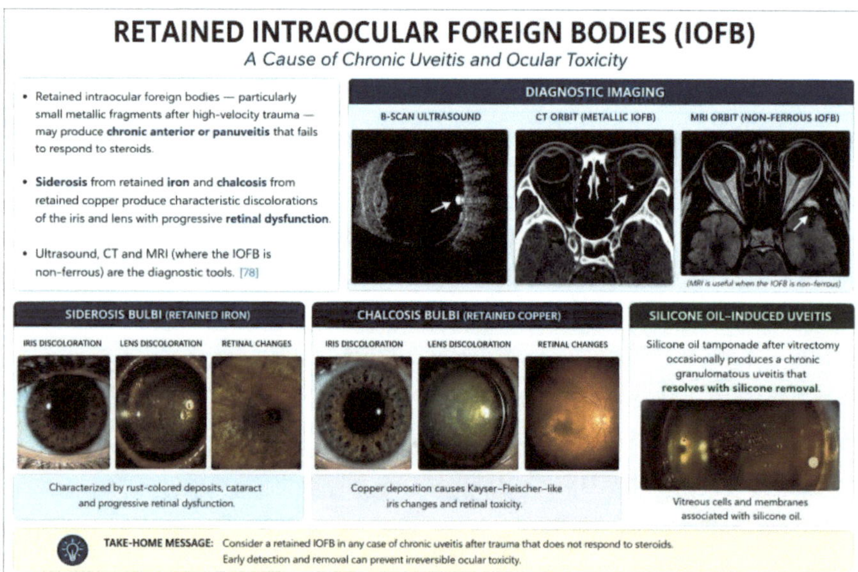

11.4 Post-surgical masquerades

Postoperative inflammation after cataract surgery is sometimes neither infectious endophthalmitis nor sterile inflammation: it may be a retained lens fragment in the vitreous, a residual capsular plaque, toxic anterior segment syndrome (TASS) from contaminated instruments, or — rarely — an indolent Propionibacterium acnes infection presenting weeks to months after surgery. Each demands a specific diagnostic and therapeutic approach.[46] The clinician should distinguish these entities before treating them as 'persistent post-operative uveitis'.

CLINICAL PEARLS

- Every uveitis history must include a complete drug review — check the recent additions.
- Rifabutin causes a bilateral hypopyon uveitis that resolves with dose reduction or discontinuation.
- MEK inhibitors produce serous retinopathy mimicking VKH/CSCR — always check OCT in oncology patients.
- Persistent postoperative uveitis after cataract surgery may be P. acnes — consider biopsy.

KEY POINTS

- Drug-induced uveitis is increasing as oncology pharmacopoeia expands.
- Recognising the offending drug is the diagnosis; co-management with the prescriber is the therapy.
- Retained IOFB and silicone oil are classic structural-iatrogenic masquerades.
- Post-surgical inflammation has multiple distinct aetiologies — never assume one cause.

SECTION III · CHAPTER 12

Rare and Paediatric Masquerades

The Atlas of the Unusual

The last chapter belongs to the rare. Some of these entities every clinician will encounter once in a career; some never. But each makes a powerful teaching point: no clinical pattern is absolute, and the eye continues to teach us through its outliers. Coats disease, persistent fetal vasculature, juvenile idiopathic arthritis with atypical phenotype, retinal vasculitis from sys…

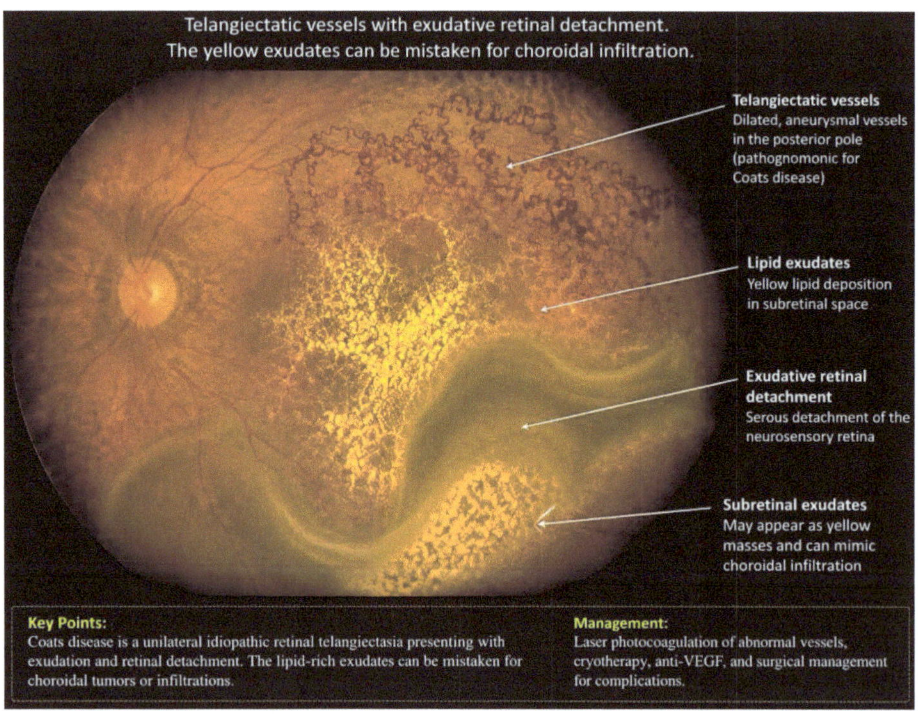

Figure 12.2 — Coats disease with telangiectatic vessels and exudative retinal detachment. The yellow exudates can be mistaken for choroidal infiltration.

CHAPTER 12

Rare and Paediatric Masquerades

The Atlas of the Unusual

The last chapter belongs to the rare. Some of these entities every clinician will encounter once in a career; some never. But each makes a powerful teaching point: no clinical pattern is absolute, and the eye continues to teach us through its outliers. Coats disease, persistent fetal vasculature, juvenile idiopathic arthritis with atypical phenotype, retinal vasculitis from systemic vasculitis, ocular ischaemic syndrome — each fills a corner of the masquerade map.[79,81,82]

12.1 Coats disease

Coats disease typically presents in young boys with unilateral telangiectatic retinal vessels and progressive exudative retinal detachment. The yellow exudates may be mistaken for choroidal infiltrates, leukaemia or retinoblastoma. B-scan ultrasound, fluorescein angiography (showing characteristic vascular abnormalities without calcification), and clinical course are diagnostic.[79,81] Treatment is laser photocoagulation or cryotherapy of telangiectatic vessels with intravitreal anti-VEGF as adjunct.

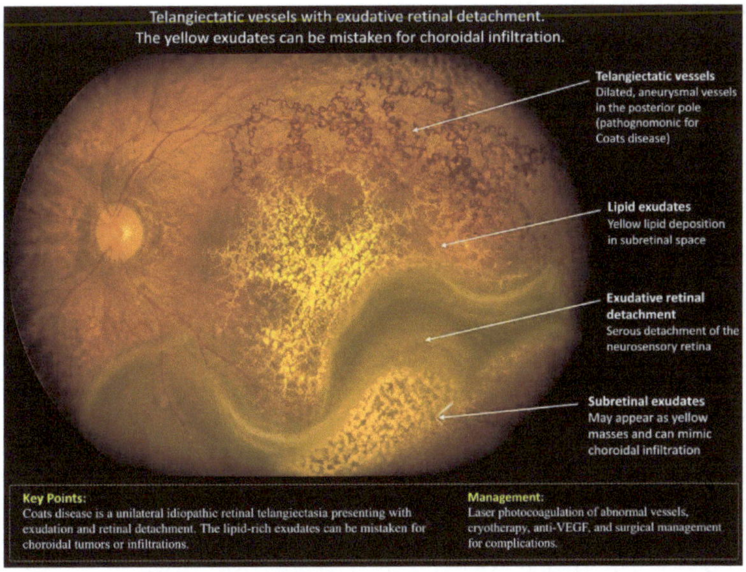

Figure 12.2 — Coats disease with telangiectatic vessels and exudative retinal detachment. The yellow exudates can be mistaken for choroidal infiltration.

12.2 Persistent fetal vasculature

Persistent fetal vasculature (PFV, formerly persistent hyperplastic primary vitreous) is a developmental anomaly presenting in infancy as leucocoria, microphthalmos, retrolental fibrovascular tissue and, in older children, recurrent vitreous haemorrhage that may be mistaken for uveitis. Diagnosis is clinical with B-scan and MRI. Early vitrectomy in selected cases can preserve some vision; the priority is to prevent amblyopia and angle-closure glaucoma.

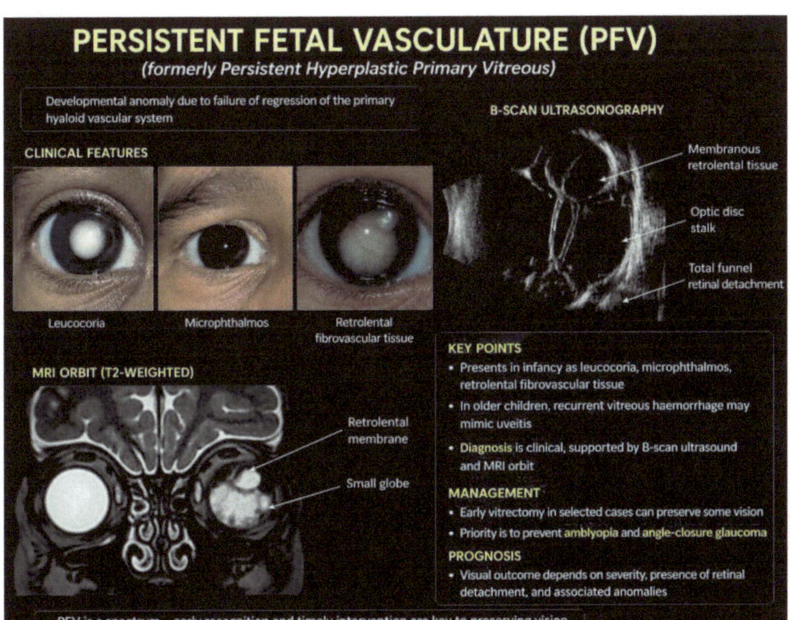

12.3 Juvenile idiopathic arthritis with atypical phenotype

Most JIA-associated uveitis is non-granulomatous, chronic and bilateral. Atypical phenotypes — granulomatous keratic precipitates, hypopyon, marked anterior chamber flare — should prompt re-evaluation. The differential includes sarcoidosis, Behçet's disease, sympathetic ophthalmia, lymphoma and tuberculosis. Periodic ophthalmic screening of every child with JIA remains a public-health priority because the majority of cases are asymptomatic until complications appear.

12.4 Ocular ischaemic syndrome

Ocular ischaemic syndrome — produced by severe carotid occlusive disease — may masquerade as chronic anterior uveitis with mid-peripheral retinal haemorrhages, narrowed retinal arterioles, and a stagnant retinal circulation. The combination of corneal oedema, low-grade cells, neovascularisation of the iris, and a paradoxically normal-appearing fundus on cursory examination should prompt carotid duplex ultrasonography.[82] Treatment is carotid revascularisation where feasible, with intraocular anti-VEGF and panretinal photocoagulation for neovascular complications.

12.5 Closing the atlas

The rare entities described here remind us that the masquerade map is never complete. New entities will be described — checkpoint-inhibitor masquerades did not exist twenty years ago — and old entities will be reframed by new science. The clinician's task is not to memorise the map but to keep redrawing it, case by case, year by year. The atlas of the unusual is the atlas of an active ophthalmologist.

CLINICAL PEARLS

- Yellow subretinal exudates in a boy with unilateral disease — think Coats, not lymphoma.
- Leucocoria in an infant with microphthalmos — think PFV, not retinoblastoma alone.
- Atypical JIA uveitis (granulomatous, hypopyon) — broaden the differential.
- Anterior uveitis with iris neovascularisation and carotid bruit — think ocular ischaemic syndrome.

KEY POINTS

- Rare entities reward the clinician who looks twice and tests broadly.
- Developmental, vascular and systemic disease can each imitate uveitis in specific contexts.
- Periodic screening of JIA is a public health intervention with proven benefit.
- The atlas of masquerade is always being redrawn — keep learning.

EPILOGUE

After the Mask Falls

We began this handbook with a patient and a question. We close it with the same. The mask of uveitis is sometimes lifted by a serology result, sometimes by an MRI, sometimes by a twenty-minute vitrectomy that returns more answers than the previous twelve months of treatment combined. But the lifting always begins with the clinician — the ophthalmologist who pauses, looks again, and asks the question that the textbook refused to write down.

There is something quietly heroic about that pause. In a discipline driven by speed and volume, the willingness to step back and reconsider is itself a clinical virtue. Every masquerade diagnosed early is a life altered, sometimes a life saved. Every masquerade missed is a slow accumulation of harm — a vitreous burdened with cells, a retina scarred by inappropriate therapy, a malignancy spreading silently while we treat the wrong diagnosis.

Ophthalmology in 2026 has never been better equipped. We have molecular cytology and high-resolution imaging that would have astonished our teachers. We have multidisciplinary tumour boards and global registries. We have the COTS studies, the SUN nomenclature, the International Workshop on Ocular Sarcoidosis criteria — a scaffolding of evidence that lets us reason in the same vocabulary across continents. The tools are unprecedented. What is required is the discipline to use them.

We hope this handbook gives you a small part of that discipline. Read it slowly the first time, mark its margins, disagree with it where you must, and keep it close. The next patient with refractory uveitis may have a malignancy hiding in their vitreous, a spirochaete swimming in their aqueous, a tumour pretending to be a cyst, or a drug quietly inflaming their iris. The faster we recognise the costume, the sooner we can treat the person underneath.

To every ophthalmologist who reads this: the mask falls when we look. May our looking be thorough, our questions persistent, and our hands gentle. The patient is depending on us.

ACKNOWLEDGMENTS

Acknowledgments

The editorial board of this handbook gratefully acknowledges the contributions of the uveitis, ocular oncology and retina services of SuVi Eye Hospital and Lasik Laser Centre, Kota. We thank our patients, who are the truest teachers of every chapter that follows; our trainees, who ask the questions that drive senior clinicians back to the textbook; and our colleagues worldwide, whose published case series, multicentre studies and case discussions have built the evidence on which this handbook rests.

We acknowledge the foundational work of the SUN Working Group, the International Workshop on Ocular Sarcoidosis, the Collaborative Ocular Tuberculosis Study (COTS), and the International Primary CNS Lymphoma Collaborative Group. The references collected in the final pages of this book are a partial repayment of that intellectual debt.

REFERENCES

References are numbered in the order of their first appearance in the text. Citations in the body of the handbook are marked with superscript numerals corresponding to this list.

1. Theodore FH. Conjunctival carcinoma masquerading as chronic conjunctivitis. Eye Ear Nose Throat Mon. 1967;46(11):1419-20.
2. Read RW, Zamir E, Rao NA. Neoplastic masquerade syndromes. Surv Ophthalmol. 2002;47(2):81-124.
3. Rothova A, Ooijman F, Kerkhoff F, Van Der Lelij A, Lokhorst HM. Uveitis masquerade syndromes. Ophthalmology. 2001;108(2):386-99.
4. Chan CC, Buggage RR, Nussenblatt RB. Intraocular lymphoma. Curr Opin Ophthalmol. 2002;13(6):411-8.
5. Chan CC, Rubenstein JL, Coupland SE, Davis JL, Harbour JW, Johnston PB, et al. Primary vitreoretinal lymphoma: a report from an International Primary Central Nervous System Lymphoma Collaborative Group symposium. Oncologist. 2011;16(11):1589-99.
6. Coupland SE, Anastassiou G, Bornfeld N, Hummel M, Stein H. Primary intraocular lymphoma of T-cell type: report of a case and review of the literature. Graefes Arch Clin Exp Ophthalmol. 2005;243(3):189-97.
7. Chan CC, Wallace DJ. Intraocular lymphoma: update on diagnosis and management. Cancer Control. 2004;11(5):285-95.
8. Whitcup SM, de Smet MD, Rubin BI, Palestine AG, Martin DF, Burnier M Jr, et al. Intraocular lymphoma. Clinical and histopathologic diagnosis. Ophthalmology. 1993;100(9):1399-406.
9. Cassoux N, Giron A, Bodaghi B, Tran TH, Baudet S, Davy F, et al. IL-10 measurement in aqueous humor for screening patients with suspicion of primary intraocular lymphoma. Invest Ophthalmol Vis Sci. 2007;48(7):3253-9.

10. Bonzheim I, Giese S, Deuter C, Süsskind D, Zierhut M, Waizel M, et al. High frequency of MYD88 mutations in vitreoretinal B-cell lymphoma: a valuable tool to improve diagnostic yield of vitreous aspirates. Blood. 2015;126(1):76-9.

11. Touhami S, Audo I, Terrada C, Gaudric A, LeHoang P, Touitou V, et al. Neoplasia and intraocular inflammation: from masquerade syndromes to immunotherapy-induced uveitis. Prog Retin Eye Res. 2019;72:100761.

12. Davis JL, Miller DM, Ruiz P. Diagnostic testing of vitrectomy specimens. Am J Ophthalmol. 2005;140(5):822-9.

13. Aronow ME, Singh AD. Diagnostic and therapeutic vitrectomy for uveitis: new analysis. Ophthalmol Eye Dis. 2014;6:51-65.

14. Rubenstein JL, Hsi ED, Johnson JL, Jung SH, Nakashima MO, Grant B, et al. Intensive chemotherapy and immunotherapy in patients with newly diagnosed primary CNS lymphoma: CALGB 50202. J Clin Oncol. 2013;31(25):3061-8.

15. Frenkel S, Hendler K, Siegal T, Shalom E, Pe'er J. Intravitreal methotrexate for treating vitreoretinal lymphoma: 10 years of experience. Br J Ophthalmol. 2008;92(3):383-8.

16. Shields JA, Shields CL, Brotman HK, Carvalho C, Perez N, Eagle RC Jr. Cancer metastatic to the orbit: the 2000 Robert M. Curts Lecture. Ophthal Plast Reconstr Surg. 2001;17(5):346-54.

17. Shields CL, Shields JA, Gross NE, Schwartz GP, Lally SE. Survey of 520 eyes with uveal metastases. Ophthalmology. 1997;104(8):1265-76.

18. Singh AD, Borden EC. Metastatic uveal melanoma. Ophthalmol Clin North Am. 2005;18(1):143-50.

19. Shields CL, Kaliki S, Furuta M, Mashayekhi A, Shields JA. Clinical spectrum and prognosis of uveal melanoma based on age at presentation in 8,033 cases. Retina. 2012;32(7):1363-72.

20. Demirci H, Shields CL, Shields JA, Honavar SG, Eagle RC Jr. Diffuse iris melanoma: a report of 25 cases. Ophthalmology. 2002;109(8):1553-60.

21. Shields JA, Shields CL. Sebaceous adenocarcinoma of the eyelid. Int Ophthalmol Clin. 2009;49(4):45-61.

22. Shields CL, Demirci H, Marr BP, Eagle RC Jr, Shields JA. Conjunctival lymphoma: clinical and prognostic features in 117 eyes. Arch Ophthalmol. 2005;123(11):1503-8.

23. Lee GA, Hirst LW. Ocular surface squamous neoplasia. Surv Ophthalmol. 1995;39(6):429-50.

24. Shields CL, Shields JA. Retinoblastoma management: advances in enucleation, intravenous chemoreduction, and intra-arterial chemotherapy. Curr Opin Ophthalmol. 2010;21(3):203-12.

25. Aziz HA, Plesec TP, Sabella MD, Manochakian R, Singh AD. Vitreoretinal lymphoma: an update. Saudi J Ophthalmol. 2015;29(2):106-12.

26. Chan CC, Sen HN. Current concepts in diagnosing and managing primary vitreoretinal (intraocular) lymphoma. Discov Med. 2013;15(81):93-100.

27. Eckardt C, Eckardt U, Groos S, Luciano L, Reale E. Removal of the internal limiting membrane in macular holes. Clinical and morphological findings. Ophthalmologe. 1997;94(8):545-51.

28. Coupland SE, Damato B. Understanding intraocular lymphomas. Clin Exp Ophthalmol. 2008;36(6):564-78.

29. Mochizuki M, Smith JR, Takase H, Kaburaki T, Acharya NR, Rao NA. Revised criteria of International Workshop on Ocular Sarcoidosis (IWOS) for the diagnosis of ocular sarcoidosis. Br J Ophthalmol. 2019;103(10):1418-22.

30. Herbort CP, Rao NA, Mochizuki M. International criteria for the diagnosis of ocular sarcoidosis: results of the first International Workshop on Ocular Sarcoidosis (IWOS). Ocul Immunol Inflamm. 2009;17(3):160-9.

31. Gupta V, Gupta A, Rao NA. Intraocular tuberculosis—an update. Surv Ophthalmol. 2007;52(6):561-87.

32. Agrawal R, Gunasekeran DV, Grant R, Agarwal A, Kon OM, Nguyen QD, et al. Clinical features and outcomes of patients with tubercular uveitis treated with antitubercular therapy in the Collaborative Ocular Tuberculosis Study (COTS-1). JAMA Ophthalmol. 2017;135(12):1318-27.

33. Furtado JM, Smith JR, Belfort R Jr, Gattey D, Winthrop KL. Toxoplasmosis: a global threat. J Glob Infect Dis. 2011;3(3):281-4.

34. Tsui E, Gonzales JA. Syphilitic uveitis. Clin Exp Ophthalmol. 2022;50(2):234-46.

35. Davis JL. Ocular syphilis. Curr Opin Ophthalmol. 2014;25(6):513-8.

36. Khairallah M, Yahia SB, Toumi A, Jelliti B, Loussaief C, Romdhane FB, et al. Severe ischemic maculopathy in a patient with West Nile virus infection. Ophthalmic Surg Lasers Imaging. 2010;41 Online:e1-3.

37. Krishnaswami V, Subbiah V, Krishnaswami A, Singh G. Ocular tuberculosis in immunocompetent and immunocompromised: a review. Curr Opin Ophthalmol. 2021;32(6):558-65.

38. Wakabayashi T, Morimura Y, Miyamoto Y, Okada AA. Changing patterns of intraocular inflammatory disease in Japan. Ocul Immunol Inflamm. 2003;11(4):277-86.

39. Stoffel M, Maeker E, Petitjean A, Wisinger C, Lefort A. IgG4-related ophthalmic disease: clinical and pathologic features. Curr Opin Ophthalmol. 2018;29(4):348-54.

40. Mahr A, Guillevin L, Poissonnet M, Aymé S. Prevalences of polyarteritis nodosa, microscopic polyangiitis, Wegener's granulomatosis, and Churg-Strauss syndrome in a French urban multiethnic population in 2000: a capture-recapture estimate. Arthritis Rheum. 2004;51(1):92-9.

41. Tarsia C, Carnevale C, Pacella E. Ocular involvement in granulomatosis with polyangiitis. Reumatismo. 2014;66(2):144-7.

42. Saw VP, Beaconsfield M, Collin JR. Conjunctival sarcoidosis: a rare cause of granulomatous conjunctivitis. Br J Ophthalmol. 2005;89(3):393-4.

43. Vasconcelos-Santos DV, Rao PK, Davies JB, Sohn EH, Rao NA. Clinical features of tuberculous serpiginous-like choroiditis in contrast to classic serpiginous choroiditis. Arch Ophthalmol. 2010;128(7):853-8.

44. Tey MS, Ng L, Choo MM. Uveitis associated with checkpoint inhibitors: a review. Clin Exp Ophthalmol. 2021;49(4):361-71.

45. Anand R, Nightingale SD, Fish RH, Smith TJ, Ashton P. Control of cytomegalovirus retinitis using sustained release of intraocular ganciclovir. Arch Ophthalmol. 1993;111(2):223-7.

46. Fardeau C, Champion E, Massamba N, LeHoang P. Uveitic macular edema. Eye (Lond). 2016;30(10):1277-92.

47. Reddy AK, Patnaik JL, Miller DC, Lynch AM, Palestine AG. Risk factors associated with persistent anterior uveitis after cataract surgery. Am J Ophthalmol. 2019;208:223-9.

48. Daniel Diaz J, Gradin D, Vrabec T, Singh AD. Diffuse anterior retinoblastoma: a diagnostic challenge. Ocul Oncol Pathol. 2017;3(3):223-7.

49. Kim JE, Patel S, Mavrofrides E, Holz ER. Bilateral retinal infiltration as the initial presenting sign of relapsed acute lymphoblastic leukemia. Retina. 2003;23(5):721-3.

50. Sharma T, Grewal J, Gupta S, Murray PI. Ophthalmic manifestations of acute leukaemias: the ophthalmologist's role. Eye (Lond). 2004;18(7):663-72.

51. Hong S, Han SB, Kim KH, Hyon JY, Lim CW, Wee WR, et al. Ocular complications of acute lymphoblastic leukemia in children: a population-based study. Korean J Ophthalmol. 2011;25(5):311-7.

52. Holz FG, Hoyng C, Ruiz Moreno JM, Bandello F. Geographic atrophy: current concepts and future avenues. Curr Opin Ophthalmol. 2020;31(4):248-54.

53. Jabs DA, Nussenblatt RB, Rosenbaum JT; Standardization of Uveitis Nomenclature (SUN) Working Group. Standardization of uveitis nomenclature for reporting clinical data. Results of the First International Workshop. Am J Ophthalmol. 2005;140(3):509-16.

54. Trusko B, Thorne J, Jabs D, Belfort R, Dick A, Gangaputra S, et al. The Standardization of Uveitis Nomenclature (SUN) Project. Development of a clinical evidence base utilizing informatics tools and techniques. Methods Inf Med. 2013;52(3):259-65.

55. Coupland SE. Molecular pathology of lymphoma. Eye (Lond). 2013;27(2):180-9.

56. Touitou V, LeHoang P, Bodaghi B. Primary intraocular lymphoma. Ophthalmologica. 2014;231(3):125-37.

57. Davis JL, Solomon D, Nussenblatt RB, Palestine AG, Chan CC. Immunocytochemical staining of vitreous cells. Indications, techniques, and results. Ophthalmology. 1992;99(2):250-6.

58. Sallam A, Taylor SR, Rajesh B, Lightman S. Indications, methods, and outcomes of vitrectomy in the diagnosis and management of uveitis. Curr Opin Ophthalmol. 2010;21(6):495-503.

59. Mochizuki M, Sugita S, Kamoi K, Takase H. A new era of uveitis: impact of polymerase chain reaction in intraocular inflammatory diseases. Jpn J Ophthalmol. 2017;61(1):1-20.

60. Sugita S, Ogawa M, Inoue Y, Takase H, Mochizuki M. Diagnosis of ocular toxoplasmosis by two polymerase chain reaction (PCR) examinations: qualitative multiplex and quantitative real-time. Jpn J Ophthalmol. 2011;55(5):495-501.

61. Drancourt M, Berger P, Raoult D. Systematic 16S rRNA gene sequencing of atypical clinical isolates identified 27 new bacterial species associated with humans. J Clin Microbiol. 2004;42(5):2197-202.

62. Karma A, Huhti E, Poukkula A. Course and outcome of ocular sarcoidosis. Am J Ophthalmol. 1988;106(4):467-72.

63. Pasadhika S, Rosenbaum JT. Ocular sarcoidosis. Clin Chest Med. 2015;36(4):669-83.

64. Birnbaum AD, Goldstein DA. Sarcoid uveitis: an update. Sarcoidosis Vasc Diffuse Lung Dis. 2012;29(2):88-95.

65. Imai A, Sugita S, Kusuhara S, Ohshita T, Mochizuki M. Molecular detection of Mycobacterium tuberculosis in cases of clinically diagnosed tuberculous uveitis. Jpn J Ophthalmol. 2015;59(2):65-72.

66. Babu RB, Sudharshan S, Kumarasamy N, Therese L, Biswas J. Ocular tuberculosis in acquired immunodeficiency syndrome. Am J Ophthalmol. 2006;142(3):413-8.

67. Bansal R, Gupta A, Gupta V, Dogra MR, Bambery P, Arora SK. Role of anti-tubercular therapy in uveitis with latent/manifest tuberculosis. Am J Ophthalmol. 2008;146(5):772-9.

68. Lou SM, Larkin KL, Winthrop K, Rosenbaum JT; Uveitis Specialists Study Group. Lessons learned from the management of refractory uveitis. Ocul Immunol Inflamm. 2014;22(5):350-7.

69. Foster CS, Vitale AT, editors. Diagnosis and treatment of uveitis. 2nd ed. New Delhi: Jaypee Brothers Medical Publishers; 2013.

70. Nussenblatt RB, Whitcup SM. Uveitis: fundamentals and clinical practice. 4th ed. Edinburgh: Mosby Elsevier; 2010.

71. Rao NA, Forster DJ, Augsburger JJ. The uvea: uveitis and intraocular neoplasms. New York: Gower Medical Publishing; 1992.

72. Maccheron LJ, Groeneveld ER, Ohlrich SJ, Hilford DJ, Beckingsale AB. Orbital lymphoproliferative disease after intense pulsed light therapy. Clin Exp Ophthalmol. 2010;38(7):734-6.

73. Patel SS, Rutzen AR, Marx JL, Thach AB, Chong LP, Rao NA. Cytomegalovirus papillitis in patients with acquired immune deficiency syndrome. Visual prognosis of patients treated with ganciclovir and/or foscarnet. Ophthalmology. 1996;103(9):1476-82.

74. Trivedi D, Denniston AK, Murray PI. Safety profile of anterior chamber paracentesis performed at the slit-lamp. Clin Exp Ophthalmol. 2011;39(8):725-8.

75. Hwang DK, Chou YJ, Pu CY, Chou P. Diagnostic vitrectomy for primary intraocular lymphoma: when, why, how? Int Ophthalmol Clin. 2014;54(2):155-71.

76. Khan KN, Mahroo OA, Khan RS, Mohamed MD, McKibbin M, Bird A, et al. Differentiating drusen: drusen and drusen-like appearances associated with ageing, age-related macular degeneration, inherited eye disease and other pathological processes. Prog Retin Eye Res. 2016;53:70-106.

77. Karkhaneh R, Lashay A, Ahmadraji A. Ocular metastasis from solid tumors: a retrospective single-center study. Iran J Ophthalmol. 2010;22(4):3-7.

78. Yonekawa Y, Kim IK. Epidemiology and management of uveal melanoma. Hematol Oncol Clin North Am. 2012;26(6):1169-84.

79. Damato BE. Tumour fluorescence and tumour-associated fluorescence of choroidal melanoma. Eye (Lond). 1992;6(Pt 6):587-93.

80. Chuck RS, Behrens A, Wellik S, Yoon J, Ngan T, Sadda S, et al. Hypertensive iridocyclitis secondary to cytomegalovirus: clinical manifestations, diagnosis, treatment, and surveillance. Curr Opin Ophthalmol. 2012;23(6):541-6.

81. Saatci AO, Ayhan Z, Engin Durmaz C, Takes O. Coats disease: a comprehensive review of literature. Open Ophthalmol J. 2014;8:18-25.

82. Shields JA, Shields CL. Differentiation of Coats' disease and retinoblastoma. J Pediatr Ophthalmol Strabismus. 2001;38(5):262-6.

83. Hayreh SS. Ocular ischemic syndrome: clinical features and management. Indian J Ophthalmol. 2014;62(11):1015-23.

84. Yanoff M, Sassani JW. Ocular pathology. 7th ed. Edinburgh: Saunders Elsevier; 2015.

85. Rao NA. Mechanisms of inflammatory response in sympathetic ophthalmia and VKH syndrome. Eye (Lond). 1997;11(Pt 2):213-6.

86. Goldberg NR, Lyu T, Moshier E, Godbold J, Jabs DA. Success with single-agent immunosuppression for multifocal choroidopathies. Am J Ophthalmol. 2014;158(6):1310-7.e1.

APPENDIX A

Glossary of Terms

A working vocabulary for the clinician at the slit lamp. Terms are listed alphabetically; cross-references to chapters appear in the Subject Index (Appendix D).

Amelanotic melanoma. A melanoma with absent or minimal pigment, often misdiagnosed as inflammatory granuloma or amelanotic metastasis.

Anterior chamber tap. Aspiration of 50-150 μL of aqueous humour from the anterior chamber for PCR or cytology in suspected infectious or neoplastic disease.

Anti-VEGF therapy. Intravitreal injection of vascular endothelial growth factor inhibitors (bevacizumab, ranibizumab, aflibercept) used to suppress neovascularisation or exudation.

ARN — Acute retinal necrosis. A fulminant viral retinitis usually caused by herpes simplex or varicella-zoster virus, presenting as panuveitis with peripheral retinitis and occlusive vasculitis.

Autofluorescence — Fundus. Imaging of the natural fluorescence of retinal pigment epithelium lipofuscin; characteristic 'leopard spotting' patterns are seen in PVRL.

BCNV — Bilateral chronic non-granulomatous vitritis. An informal label often applied to PVRL before diagnosis.

CAR — Cancer-associated retinopathy. A paraneoplastic autoimmune retinopathy producing photopsia and progressive visual loss, typically associated with small-cell lung carcinoma.

Carrier-state TB. Latent tuberculosis identified by IGRA positivity without active disease; relevant when considering anti-tubercular therapy in suspected ocular TB.

Choroidal granuloma. A discrete dome-shaped or plateau-shaped infiltrative lesion of the choroid seen in sarcoidosis, TB, syphilis or lymphoma.

Choroidal metastasis. Haematogenous deposit in the choroid from a distant primary malignancy; most common adult intraocular tumour overall.

Cidofovir uveitis. Anterior uveitis with hypotony induced by intravenous or intravitreal cidofovir in the management of CMV retinitis.

CME — Cystoid macular oedema. Cystic intraretinal fluid accumulation, frequently complicating uveitis and masquerade syndromes.

CNS-relapse. Recurrence of primary CNS lymphoma in the central nervous system after initial remission.

Coats disease. A unilateral retinal vascular telangiectasia of unknown cause, typically affecting young boys with exudative retinal detachment.

Cytology — Vitreous. Microscopic examination of cells obtained by vitreous biopsy; pillar of PVRL diagnosis.

Diffuse iris melanoma. A flat infiltrative iris melanoma producing heterochromia and pigment dispersion, often misdiagnosed as glaucoma.

EDI-OCT. Enhanced-depth imaging OCT for assessment of choroidal thickness, used in VKH and inflammatory choroidopathies.

Endogenous endophthalmitis. Infection of the eye arising from haematogenous spread of bacteria or fungi from a distant focus.

Endotheliitis — Corneal. Endothelial inflammation with associated keratic precipitates, often caused by CMV in immunocompetent adults.

Eales disease. Idiopathic peripheral retinal vasculitis with neovascularisation, classically described in young Indian men and often associated with TB sensitisation.

ERG — Electroretinogram. Recording of the electrical response of retinal cells to light stimulation; essential in paraneoplastic retinopathy diagnosis.

FAF — Fundus autofluorescence. Functional imaging used to detect RPE-level abnormalities.

FFA — Fundus fluorescein angiography. Imaging of retinal and choroidal vasculature using intravenous sodium fluorescein.

Flow cytometry. Cell-by-cell analysis of immunophenotype, used to detect monoclonal B-cell populations in PVRL.

Foreign body — IOFB. Any retained intraocular foreign material, commonly metallic, that may produce chronic uveitis or siderosis.

FTA-ABS / TPHA. Treponemal-specific syphilis serology tests.

GPA — Granulomatosis with polyangiitis. ANCA-associated systemic vasculitis with ocular manifestations including necrotising scleritis and peripheral ulcerative keratitis.

HFUS / UBM. High-frequency ultrasound / ultrasound biomicroscopy used to image anterior segment structures and iridociliary masses.

HRCT — High-resolution chest CT. Imaging used to screen for pulmonary sarcoidosis, tuberculosis or interstitial disease in ocular masquerade workup.

ICG — Indocyanine green angiography. Imaging of choroidal vasculature; hypofluorescent dark spots are characteristic of lymphomatous infiltration.

IgG4-related disease. A systemic fibroinflammatory disorder with characteristic IgG4-positive plasma cell infiltrate, producing orbital and ophthalmic disease.

IGRA — Interferon-gamma release assay. Blood test for tuberculosis sensitisation; the COTS studies have established its place in ocular TB diagnosis.

IL-10:IL-6 ratio. Vitreous cytokine ratio greater than 1.0 supports the diagnosis of primary vitreoretinal lymphoma.

Immune-checkpoint inhibitor uveitis. Uveitis or VKH-like syndrome induced by ipilimumab, nivolumab or pembrolizumab.

IRBP — Interphotoreceptor retinoid-binding protein. Retinal autoantigen targeted in some paraneoplastic retinopathies.

Iris nodules. Stromal or pupillary nodules seen in granulomatous uveitis (sarcoid, TB) and iris melanoma.

JIA — Juvenile idiopathic arthritis. Chronic paediatric arthritis with associated chronic anterior uveitis; periodic screening is mandatory.

Leucocoria. A white pupillary reflex; in children, an urgent sign for retinoblastoma, PFV, Coats and other retinal pathology.

Limbal mass. Lesion at the corneoscleral junction; differential includes OSSN, conjunctival melanoma, lymphoma and pterygium with atypia.

Lymphoid follicle. Reactive lymphoid aggregate seen on biopsy; must be distinguished from monoclonal lymphoma.

MAR — Melanoma-associated retinopathy. Paraneoplastic autoimmune retinopathy in cutaneous melanoma producing characteristic negative ERG.

MALT lymphoma. Mucosa-associated lymphoid tissue lymphoma; the most common conjunctival lymphoma.

MEK inhibitor retinopathy. Bilateral serous retinal detachments produced by trametinib or cobimetinib, mimicking VKH or CSCR.

Methotrexate — Intravitreal. Standard local therapy for primary vitreoretinal lymphoma at 400 μg per injection.

Mutton-fat KPs. Large greasy keratic precipitates on the corneal endothelium typical of granulomatous anterior uveitis.

MYD88 L265P. Somatic mutation present in 70-90% of primary vitreoretinal lymphomas; a near-pathognomonic molecular marker.

Necrotising scleritis. Severe scleral inflammation with tissue necrosis, often associated with systemic vasculitis.

Neuroretinitis. Optic disc swelling with peripapillary macular star, classically associated with cat-scratch disease and other infections.

OCT — Optical coherence tomography. Cross-sectional retinal imaging; the workhorse of modern uveitis practice.

OSSN — Ocular surface squamous neoplasia. Spectrum of dysplasia to invasive squamous carcinoma at the corneoscleral limbus.

Pagetoid spread. Intra-epithelial spread of sebaceous gland carcinoma along conjunctival or eyelid epithelium.

Paraneoplastic retinopathy. Autoimmune retinopathy induced by antibodies cross-reacting between tumour antigens and retinal proteins.

Pars planitis. Idiopathic intermediate uveitis with vitreous snowbanking; a diagnosis of exclusion after masquerade screen.

PCR — Polymerase chain reaction. Molecular detection of viral, bacterial or parasitic DNA from aqueous or vitreous samples.

PFV — Persistent fetal vasculature. Developmental anomaly with retrolental fibrovascular tissue; presents with leucocoria in infants.

PIOL / PVRL. Primary intraocular lymphoma / primary vitreoretinal lymphoma.

PORN — Progressive outer retinal necrosis. Fulminant VZV retinitis in profound immunocompromise.

Posner-Schlossman syndrome. Recurrent unilateral hypertensive anterior uveitis; CMV is a frequent cause.

Posterior placoid chorioretinitis. Yellow placoid macular lesion characteristic of acute syphilitic posterior chorioretinitis.

Pseudo-hypopyon. A layered cellular deposit in the anterior chamber that may be lymphomatous, leukaemic, or sebaceous gland carcinoma cells, not always inflammatory.

Retinoblastoma — Diffuse infiltrating. A variant of retinoblastoma producing vitritis and pseudo-hypopyon, classically in children aged 3-7 years.

Rifabutin uveitis. Bilateral hypopyon uveitis induced by rifabutin, dose-related and reversible on discontinuation.

Roth spot. Retinal haemorrhage with white centre, classical in leukaemia, endocarditis and other haematological disease.

Sarcoid uveitis. Granulomatous panuveitis, intermediate uveitis or anterior uveitis associated with systemic sarcoidosis.

Sebaceous gland carcinoma. Lethal eyelid carcinoma mimicking chalazion and chronic blepharitis.

Sentinel vessel. Dilated episcleral vessel marking the location of an underlying ciliary body tumour.

Serpiginous-like choroiditis. TB-related multifocal serpiginous choroiditis distinct from classic idiopathic serpiginous choroiditis.

SUN — Standardisation of Uveitis Nomenclature. International consensus framework for uveitis classification and reporting.

Sympathetic ophthalmia. Bilateral granulomatous panuveitis following penetrating ocular injury or surgery to the fellow eye.

TASS — Toxic anterior segment syndrome. Acute sterile postoperative inflammation following cataract surgery, mimicking endophthalmitis.

Trametinib retinopathy. Serous retinal detachments produced by MEK inhibitor trametinib.

Tuberculin skin test. Mantoux skin test for TB sensitisation, less commonly used than IGRA in modern practice.

Uveal melanoma. The most common primary intraocular malignancy in adults; the iris, ciliary body and choroid are all potential sites.

VDRL / RPR. Non-treponemal syphilis serology tests.

Visual prognosis — Late masquerade. Late diagnosis of masquerade syndromes is associated with worse visual outcomes and higher mortality where neoplastic.

Vitreous biopsy. Surgical sampling of vitreous for cytology, flow cytometry, cytokines and molecular tests; the procedural cornerstone of PVRL diagnosis.

VKH — Vogt-Koyanagi-Harada. Bilateral granulomatous panuveitis with neurological, auditory and integumentary features.

Whipple disease. Rare systemic infection by Tropheryma whipplei with chronic vitritis and retinitis among ocular manifestations.

Xanthogranuloma — Juvenile. Histiocytic infiltration of the iris in young children, producing spontaneous hyphaema.

APPENDIX B

Clinical Case Vignettes

Five vignettes drawn from the everyday work of the masquerade clinic. Each ends with a single teaching point that the editors would defend in any clinical conversation.

CASE VIGNETTE

Case 1 — The 72-year-old with 'refractory intermediate uveitis'

PRESENTATION

A 72-year-old retired teacher was referred with 14 months of bilateral, asymmetric vitritis that had been treated with topical, periocular and oral corticosteroids without sustained improvement. Visual acuity was 6/24 in the right eye and 6/18 in the left. Both eyes had vitreous cells in clumps and sheets, with subtle yellowish subretinal deposits at the macula.

INVESTIGATIONS

OCT showed hyper-reflective sub-RPE deposits with RPE undulations. Fundus autofluorescence demonstrated a granular 'leopard' pattern. MRI of the brain revealed periventricular enhancement. Diagnostic vitrectomy of the right eye returned cytology positive for atypical lymphoid cells with high N:C ratio, MYD88 L265P mutation positive, and IL-10:IL-6 ratio of 8.4. CSF cytology confirmed CNS involvement.

DIAGNOSIS

Primary vitreoretinal lymphoma with CNS involvement (PVRL/PCNSL).

MANAGEMENT

Intravitreal methotrexate (400 μg) weekly for 4 weeks induction, twice-weekly consolidation and monthly maintenance. Systemic high-dose methotrexate-based chemotherapy initiated by the haematology-oncology team. Surveillance MRI brain at 3 months.

TEACHING POINT

Bilateral steroid-resistant vitritis in an adult over 60 years is PVRL until proven otherwise. OCT and FAF often suggest the diagnosis before cytology returns.

CASE VIGNETTE

Case 2 — The 38-year-old with 'recurrent anterior uveitis'

PRESENTATION

A 38-year-old man presented with three episodes of anterior uveitis over 8 months. Each episode partially responded to topical steroids but recurred within weeks of taper. Vision remained 6/9 in both eyes. He admitted to multiple sexual partners over the last two years.

INVESTIGATIONS

Tier-1 masquerade screen: VDRL reactive at 1:64, FTA-ABS positive. HIV serology negative. CSF examination demonstrated reactive VDRL and lymphocytic pleocytosis.

DIAGNOSIS

Ocular syphilis with neurosyphilis.

MANAGEMENT

Intravenous benzylpenicillin 4 million units every 4 hours for 14 days, with public health notification and partner-tracing. Visual acuity normalised within 4 weeks and inflammation did not recur.

TEACHING POINT

Every undifferentiated uveitis must have syphilis serology checked. The 'new great imitator' responds dramatically to neurosyphilis-protocol penicillin.

CASE VIGNETTE

Case 3 — The 4-year-old with 'persistent uveitis'

PRESENTATION

A 4-year-old boy was referred with a 6-month history of unilateral pseudo-hypopyon and vitritis treated with topical corticosteroids. The fellow eye was normal. Family had noted occasional 'cat's eye' reflex in photographs.

INVESTIGATIONS

Examination under anaesthesia revealed pseudo-hypopyon with vitreous seeds. B-scan ultrasound demonstrated calcification within a vitreous mass. MRI orbits and brain confirmed an intraocular tumour without extraocular extension or pinealoma.

DIAGNOSIS

Diffuse infiltrating retinoblastoma.

MANAGEMENT

Enucleation with long optic nerve resection, histopathology confirmed retinoblastoma with no extraocular extension. Adjuvant chemotherapy was initially planned but, given clear margins, deferred per multidisciplinary tumour-board decision. Genetic counselling provided.

TEACHING POINT

Any unilateral uveitis in a child under 7 demands retinoblastoma exclusion. Vitreous biopsy is contraindicated. EUA, B-scan and MRI are the diagnostic triad.

CASE VIGNETTE

Case 4 — The 56-year-old breast cancer survivor with 'choroidal effusion'

PRESENTATION

A 56-year-old woman with a 4-year history of treated breast cancer (in clinical remission) presented with sudden visual blurring in the right eye. Examination revealed a creamy yellow choroidal lesion 2 disc-diameters in size with overlying serous retinal detachment.

INVESTIGATIONS

B-scan: moderately reflective lesion, 3.2 mm thick, with low internal reflectivity. OCT: dome elevation with subretinal fluid. ICG: discrete hypofluorescent mass. Systemic restaging with CT/PET demonstrated hepatic and bone metastases.

DIAGNOSIS

Choroidal metastasis from breast carcinoma, heralding systemic relapse.

MANAGEMENT

External beam radiotherapy 25 Gy in 10 fractions to the right eye with concurrent systemic chemotherapy. Intravitreal anti-VEGF for the secondary serous detachment. Choroidal lesion regressed at 3-month follow-up.

TEACHING POINT

Choroidal metastasis frequently announces a systemic relapse in cancer survivors. Urgent oncology referral is part of the ophthalmic management.

CASE VIGNETTE

Case 5 — The 64-year-old on trametinib with 'sudden VKH-like uveitis'

PRESENTATION

A 64-year-old man on trametinib for metastatic cutaneous melanoma presented with bilateral blurred vision, mild headache, and no anterior segment inflammation. OCT demonstrated bilateral multifocal serous retinal detachments.

INVESTIGATIONS

Choroidal thickness on EDI-OCT was mildly increased. ICG showed minimal abnormality. Investigations for VKH (HLA-DR4 typing, neurological assessment, audiogram) were non-contributory. Drug review confirmed recent introduction of trametinib.

DIAGNOSIS

MEK-inhibitor (trametinib) retinopathy.

MANAGEMENT

Co-management with the medical oncology team. Trametinib was held briefly with rapid resolution of the serous detachments. Restarted at a reduced dose with regular OCT monitoring. No oral steroids required.

TEACHING POINT

Bilateral serous retinal detachments in an oncology patient must trigger a drug review before a VKH workup. MEK inhibitor retinopathy resolves on dose reduction.

APPENDIX C

Diagnostic Checklist for the Daily Uveitis Clinic

A short, deliberately repetitive checklist for the first visit of any patient with apparent uveitis. It is meant to be photocopied and kept beside the slit lamp. Two extra minutes per patient may save twelve months of inappropriate therapy.

HISTORY

Onset, laterality, duration, prior treatments, response, current medications (with specific attention to recent additions), comorbidities (cancer, autoimmune, immunocompromise), travel, sexual history, constitutional symptoms.

EXAMINATION

External lids, conjunctiva, sclera, cornea, anterior chamber cells and flare, iris stromal detail and nodules, IOP, gonioscopy if pigment dispersion, lens, vitreous cells (discrete vs clumped), full dilated fundus examination with peripheral retina.

IMAGING

OCT macula and disc, fundus autofluorescence, fundus photograph, FFA / ICG if posterior involvement, B-scan if media opacity, HFUS/UBM if iridociliary process suspected, anterior segment OCT if surface lesion.

TIER-1 SYSTEMIC SCREEN (ALWAYS)

VDRL/RPR + treponemal (FTA-ABS or TPHA), HIV, CBC + peripheral smear, ESR, CRP, ACE, lysozyme, chest X-ray ± HRCT, IGRA in endemic regions or risk factors.

TIER-2 (SELECTED)

ANCA, ANA, dsDNA, complement, serum IgG4, MRI brain/orbits, lumbar puncture with CSF cytology if neoplastic suspicion, electrocardiogram, audiogram if VKH suspected.

TIER-3 (WHEN MASQUERADE SUSPECTED)

Anterior chamber tap with PCR (HSV/VZV/CMV/T. gondii); diagnostic vitrectomy with cytology, flow cytometry, IL-10:IL-6, MYD88 L265P, microbial panel; biopsy of accessible extraocular tissues; multidisciplinary tumour or infectious diseases board.

DOCUMENTATION

Photograph or detailed drawing of the eye at every visit, recorded OCT, structured notes with SUN nomenclature where applicable.

THERAPY GATE

Do not escalate steroids without re-examining the differential. Treatment failure is itself a diagnostic finding.

APPENDIX D

Subject Index

A compact subject index for navigating the handbook by clinical theme.

APPENDIX E

List of Figures, Tables and Flowcharts

A compendium of every visual element in this handbook, for quick navigation.

FIGURES

FIG_1_1 · Figure 1.1 — Slit-lamp examination is the first instrument of unmasking. The clinician's discipline, more than the lamp itself, determines what is found.

FIG_1_2 · Figure 1.2 — A library of ophthalmic literature on uveitis and masquerade syndromes, illustrating the evolving conceptual landscape since Theodore's 1967 description.

FIG_2_1 · Figure 2.1 — Cytology preparation stained with Giemsa: pleomorphic lymphoid cells with prominent nucleoli, suspicious for primary vitreoretinal lymphoma.

FIG_2_2 · Figure 2.2 — Diagnostic workflow visualised in a clinical setting. Pattern recognition across age, laterality, and treatment response forms the backbone of suspicion.

FIG_3_1 · Figure 3.1 — History-taking in a structured uveitis consultation: posterior segment masquerades are often diagnosed at the bedside before the first investigation.

FIG_3_2 · Figure 3.2 — A child with chronic anterior segment inflammation. In any uveitis under three years of age, retinoblastoma must be excluded before steroids are escalated.

FIG_4_1 · Figure 4.1 — Spectral-domain OCT illustration of subretinal hyper-reflective deposits — a clue that may signal primary vitreoretinal lymphoma rather than posterior uveitis.

FIG_4_2 · Figure 4.2 — Diagnostic vitrectomy in progress. Sample volume, handling, and rapid transit to the laboratory are the three commandments of cytological yield.

FIG_5_1 · Figure 5.1 — Vitreous cells in clumps and sheets — the 'aurora borealis' of primary vitreoretinal lymphoma seen on indirect ophthalmoscopy.

FIG_5_2 · Figure 5.2 — MRI brain coronal section showing periventricular enhancement in a patient with primary CNS lymphoma — the cerebral counterpart of the vitreoretinal disease.

FIG_6_1 · Figure 6.1 — Choroidal metastasis from breast carcinoma: a creamy, dome-shaped lesion with overlying serous detachment. Often the first sign of relapse.

FIG_6_2 · Figure 6.2 — Systemic oncology assessment. Choroidal metastasis frequently demands urgent staging, particularly in lung, breast, and gastrointestinal primaries.

FIG_7_1 · Figure 7.1 — Diffuse iris melanoma presenting as unilateral heterochromia and 'pigment dispersion glaucoma'. The pigment was the tumour.

FIG_7_2 · Figure 7.2 — High-frequency ultrasound biomicroscopy of an iridociliary cyst that had been treated for two years as recurrent anterior uveitis.

FIG_8_1 · Figure 8.1 — Ocular surface squamous neoplasia at the limbus with leukoplakic, vascularised, gelatinous appearance — initially treated for years as chronic conjunctivitis.

FIG_8_2 · Figure 8.2 — Paediatric retinal examination under anaesthesia. In any unilateral white pupil or atypical uveitis below three years of age, retinoblastoma must be excluded.

FIG_9_1 · Figure 9.1 — Ocular syphilis, the 'new great imitator', can present as anterior uveitis, posterior placoid chorioretinitis, optic neuritis or panuveitis. Serology is mandatory in every undifferentiated uveitis.

FIG_9_2 · Figure 9.2 — Chest radiograph showing apical fibrocavitary changes in a patient with ocular tuberculosis presenting as serpiginous-like choroiditis.

FIG_10_1 · Figure 10.1 — High-resolution CT chest demonstrating bilateral hilar lymphadenopathy. Ocular sarcoidosis often whispers from the chest before it shouts from the eye.

FIG_10_2 · Figure 10.2 — IgG4-related dacryoadenitis with bilateral lacrimal gland enlargement. Histopathology with IgG4+ plasma cell counts is diagnostic.

FIG_11_1 · Figure 11.1 — Drug review is part of the uveitis examination. Rifabutin, bisphosphonates, MEK and checkpoint inhibitors are common precipitants of drug-induced uveitis.

FIG_11_2 · Figure 11.2 — Retained intraocular foreign body discovered on ultrasound after months of treatment for chronic anterior uveitis — a classic iatrogenic masquerade.

TABLES

FLOWCHARTS

EDITORIAL

About the Editorial Board

The editorial board of the Masquerade Syndrome Clinical Handbook brings together ophthalmologists, uveitis specialists, ocular oncologists and trainees from the uveitis, retina and ocular oncology services of SuVi Eye Hospital and Lasik Laser Centre, Kota. The handbook was conceived in the busy outpatient clinic, drafted across morning rounds and evening tutorials, and refined through case-by-case discussion with colleagues across India and abroad.

EDITORIAL CHAIR

Senior Consultant — Uveitis & Ocular Inflammation

Three decades of clinical practice in anterior, posterior and panuveitis, with a particular interest in the diagnostic boundary between inflammation and malignancy.

OCULAR ONCOLOGY EDITOR

Consultant — Ocular Oncology & Vitreoretinal Surgery

Clinical lead for the regional vitreoretinal lymphoma service, contributor to multidisciplinary tumour boards, and an advocate for early diagnostic vitrectomy.

INFECTIOUS DISEASE EDITOR

Consultant — Uveitis & Ocular Infections

Focus on ocular syphilis, ocular tuberculosis and emerging viral retinitides; member of the regional COTS working group on tubercular uveitis.

PAEDIATRIC EDITOR

Consultant — Paediatric Ophthalmology & Strabismus

Specialist in childhood uveitis, retinoblastoma surveillance and developmental anomalies of the posterior segment.

TRAINEE EDITOR

Fellow — Uveitis Service

Curator of the case-vignette appendix and editorial proofreader; an early-career voice to ensure the handbook remains accessible to ophthalmic trainees.

ABOUT THE INSTITUTION

SuVi Eye Hospital and Lasik Laser Centre, Kota, is a comprehensive tertiary eye-care centre serving south-eastern Rajasthan and the surrounding states. Its uveitis, retina and ocular oncology services run integrated outpatient clinics, surgical lists and academic meetings. Clinical philosophy at SuVi is summarised in three habits: examine slowly, write what you see, and never escalate therapy without re-examining the diagnosis.

FURTHER STUDY

Recommended Reading and Further Study

FOUNDATIONAL TEXTBOOKS

- Nussenblatt RB, Whitcup SM. Uveitis: Fundamentals and Clinical Practice. 4th edition. Mosby Elsevier, 2010.
- Foster CS, Vitale AT (eds). Diagnosis and Treatment of Uveitis. 2nd edition. Jaypee Brothers, 2013.
- Shields JA, Shields CL. Intraocular Tumours: An Atlas and Textbook. 3rd edition. Wolters Kluwer, 2016.
- Rao NA, Forster DJ, Augsburger JJ. The Uvea: Uveitis and Intraocular Neoplasms. Gower Medical, 1992.
- Yanoff M, Sassani JW. Ocular Pathology. 7th edition. Saunders Elsevier, 2015.

LANDMARK JOURNAL ARTICLES

- Read RW, Zamir E, Rao NA. Neoplastic masquerade syndromes. Surv Ophthalmol 2002;47(2):81-124.
- Rothova A et al. Uveitis masquerade syndromes. Ophthalmology 2001;108(2):386-99.
- Chan CC et al. Primary vitreoretinal lymphoma: a report from an International Primary CNS Lymphoma Collaborative Group symposium. Oncologist 2011;16(11):1589-99.
- Bonzheim I et al. High frequency of MYD88 mutations in vitreoretinal B-cell lymphoma. Blood 2015;126(1):76-9.
- Touhami S et al. Neoplasia and intraocular inflammation. Prog Retin Eye Res 2019;72:100761.

ONLINE RESOURCES AND SOCIETIES

- International Uveitis Study Group (IUSG) — guidelines and educational meetings.
- American Uveitis Society — online case archive and tutorials.
- Standardization of Uveitis Nomenclature (SUN) Working Group — nomenclature resources.
- Collaborative Ocular Tuberculosis Study (COTS) — open-access study protocols.
- International Society for Ocular Oncology (ISOO) — guidelines for vitreoretinal lymphoma and uveal melanoma.

SUGGESTED STUDY PATH FOR THE TRAINEE

- Begin with Section I of this handbook and Theodore's 1967 paper.
- Move to PVRL by reading Chapter 5 and the Bonzheim 2015 and Chan 2011 papers.
- Read Chapter 9 alongside the most recent COTS publication and a current review on ocular syphilis.
- Use the case vignettes (Appendix B) as a self-test before each masquerade clinic.
- Build a personal scrapbook of difficult cases — photograph, OCT, outcome — over the first three years of practice.

CITATION

Citation Guidance

Editorial Board, SuVi Eye Hospital and Lasik Laser Centre, Kota. Masquerade Syndrome in Ophthalmology: A Clinical Handbook of the Great Imitators of the Eye. First Edition. Kota: SuVi Editorial Press; 2026.

If you cite a specific chapter, please name the chapter in your reference. Example: Editorial Board. Primary Vitreoretinal Lymphoma and CNS Lymphoma. In: Masquerade Syndrome in Ophthalmology. 1st ed. Kota: SuVi Editorial Press; 2026. Chapter 5.

DISCLAIMER

Disclaimer and Scope of Use

This handbook is an educational reference for qualified ophthalmologists, ophthalmic trainees and clinicians involved in the care of patients with intraocular inflammation. It is not a substitute for clinical judgement, specialist consultation, or the most current published literature.

The editorial board has made every reasonable effort to ensure that the clinical information presented reflects accepted practice at the time of writing (2026). Ophthalmic practice, particularly in the realm of molecular diagnostics and targeted therapy, evolves rapidly; clinicians are urged to consult the most recent guidelines and primary literature before making management decisions.

Doses, drug regimens and procedural protocols cited in this handbook are illustrative. Final therapeutic decisions must be tailored to the individual patient, in consultation with the multidisciplinary team where appropriate, and in accordance with local regulatory approvals.

No part of this handbook constitutes medical advice for any individual patient. The editorial board, SuVi Eye Hospital and Lasik Laser Centre, Kota, and the contributors named herein accept no liability for clinical decisions made by readers in reliance upon its content.

Colophon

MASQUERADE SYNDROME IN OPHTHALMOLOGY
First Edition · 2026
SuVi Eye Hospital and Lasik Laser Centre, Kota
Kota, Rajasthan, India

Typeset for digital and print reading.

www.ingramcontent.com/pod-product-compliance
Lightning Source LLC
LaVergne TN
LVHW070936210926
848482LV00003B/252

* 9 7 9 8 9 0 5 6 0 7 5 7 8 *